Achieving Mental Health Equity

Editors

ALTHA J. STEWART
RUTH S. SHIM

PSYCHIATRIC CLINICS
OF NORTH AMERICA

www.psych.theclinics.com

Consulting Editor
HARSH K. TRIVEDI

September 2020 • Volume 43 • Number 3

ELSEVIER

1600 John F. Kennedy Boulevard • Suite 1800 • Philadelphia, Pennsylvania, 19103-2899

http://www.theclinics.com

PSYCHIATRIC CLINICS OF NORTH AMERICA Volume 43, Number 3
September 2020 ISSN 0193-953X, ISBN-13: 978-0-323-75812-3

Editor: Lauren Boyle
Developmental Editor: Nicole Congleton

Psychiatric Clinics of North America (ISSN 0193-953X) is published quarterly by Elsevier Inc., 360 Park Avenue South, New York, NY 10010-1710. Months of issue are March, June, September, and December. Business and Editorial Offices: 1600 John F. Kennedy Blvd., Suite 1800, Philadelphia, PA 19103-2899. Periodicals postage paid at New York, NY and additional mailing offices. Subscription prices are $335.00 per year (US individuals), $734.00 per year (US institutions), $100.00 per year (US students/residents), $406.00 per year (Canadian individuals), $462.00 per year (international individuals), $924.00 per year (Canadian & international institutions), and $220.00 per year (international students/residents), $100.00 per year (Canadian & students/residents). Foreign air speed delivery is included in all *Clinics'* subscription prices. All prices are subject to change without notice. **POSTMASTER:** Send address changes to *Psychiatric Clinics of North America*, Elsevier Health Sciences Division, Subscription Customer Service, 3251 Riverport Lane, Maryland Heights, MO 63043. **Customer Service: 1-800-654-2452 (US). From outside the United States, call 1-314-447-8871. Fax: 1-314-447-8029. E-mail: journalscustomerservice-usa@elsevier.com (for print support) and journalsonlinesupport-usa@elsevier.com (for online support).**

Reprints. For copies of 100 or more, of articles in this publication, please contact the Commercial Reprints Department, Elsevier Inc., 360 Park Avenue South, New York, New York 10010-1710. Tel.: 212-633-3874, Fax: 212-633-3820, E-mail: reprints@elsevier.com.

Psychiatric Clinics of North America is covered in *MEDLINE/PubMed (Index Medicus)*, *Current Contents/Social and Behavioral Sciences, Social Science Citation Index, Embase/Excerpta Medica,* and PsycINFO.

Contributors

CONSULTING EDITOR

HARSH K. TRIVEDI, MD, MBA
President and Chief Executive Officer, Sheppard Pratt Health System, Baltimore, Maryland

EDITORS

ALTHA J. STEWART, MD
Senior Associate Dean for Community Health Engagement, Associate Professor/Chief of Social and Public Psychiatry, Director, Center for Health in Justice involved Youth, The University of Tennessee Health Science Center, Memphis, Tennessee

RUTH S. SHIM, MD, MPH
Luke and Grace Kim Professor in Cultural Psychiatry, Professor in Clinical Psychiatry, Department of Psychiatry and Behavioral Sciences, University of California, Davis, Sacramento, California

AUTHORS

CHERYL S. AL-MATEEN, MD
Professor, Departments of Psychiatry and Pediatrics, Medical Director, Virginia Treatment Center for Children, Virginia Commonwealth University, Richmond, Virginia

JEAN-MARIE ALVES-BRADFORD, MD
Associate Clinical Professor of Psychiatry, Columbia Department of Psychiatry, Associate Clinical Director and Director of the Washington Heights Community Service, New York State Psychiatric Institute, New York, New York

BRIGITTE BAILEY, MD
Professor of Psychiatry and Pediatrics, Program Director, Child and Adolescent Psychiatry, Department of Psychiatry and Behavioral Sciences, UT Health San Antonio, San Antonio, Texas

ERAKA BATH, MD
Director, Child Forensic Services, Associate Professor, Department of Psychiatry, Vice Chair for Equity, Diversity and Inclusion, UCLA Jane & Terry Semel Institute for Neuroscience & Human Behavior, Los Angeles, California

JOSEPH R. BETANCOURT, MD, MPH
Vice President, Chief Equity and Inclusion Officer, Equity and Inclusion Administration, Massachusetts General Hospital, Associate Professor of Medicine, Harvard Medical School, Boston, Massachusetts

TIMOTHY T. COFFEY, MS
Project Coordinator, Eleventh Judicial Circuit of Florida, Criminal Mental Health Project, Miami, Florida

PAMELA Y. COLLINS, MD, MPH
Professor, Departments of Psychiatry and Behavioral Sciences, and Global Health, University of Washington School of Medicine and Public Health, Seattle, Washington

ANGELA COOMBS, MD
Instructor in Clinical Psychiatry, Columbia Department of Psychiatry, Medical Director, OnTrackNY-Washington Heights Community Service

JAMES CORBETT, MDiv, JD
Principal, Initium Health, EO Health, Denver, Colorado

SANDRA M. DeJONG, MD, MSc
Assistant Professor of Psychiatry, Harvard Medical School, Senior Consultant to Child/Adolescent Psychiatry Training, Cambridge Health Alliance, Cambridge, Massachusetts

JACQUELINE MAUS FELDMAN, MD
Professor Emerita, Department of Psychiatry and Behavioral Neurobiology, The University of Alabama at Birmingham, Birmingham, Alabama

LISA R. FORTUNA, MD, MPH
Chief of Psychiatry, Zuckerberg San Francisco General Hospital and Trauma Center, Vice Chair of Psychiatry, University of California, San Francisco, San Francisco, California

SIDNEY H. HANKERSON, MD, MBA
Assistant Professor of Clinical Psychiatry, Columbia University, Vagelos College of Physicians and Surgeons, Research Scientist, New York State Psychiatric Institute, New York, New York

TOI BLAKLEY HARRIS, MD
Professor, Menninger Department of Psychiatry and Behavioral Sciences, Pediatrics, Family and Community Medicine, Associate Provost, Institutional Diversity, Inclusion and Equity and Student and Trainee Services, Center of Excellence in Health Equity, Training and Research, PI/PD, Baylor College of Medicine, Houston, Texas

JESSICA ISOM, MD, MPH
Attending Physician, Codman Square Health Center, Boston Medical Center, Dorchester, Massachusetts

NICOLE JACKSON, DSW
Forensic Mental Health Consultant, Lorio Forensics, Atlanta, Georgia

MAGA E. JACKSON-TRICHE, MD, MSHS
HSC Professor and Vice Chair for Adult Psychiatry, Vice President for Adult Behavioral Health Services, UCSF Health, UCSF Weill Institute for Neurosciences, San Francisco, California

AYANA JORDAN, MD, PhD
Assistant Professor, Department of Psychiatry, Yale School of Medicine, New Haven, Connecticut

RUPINDER KAUR LEGHA, MD
Assistant Research Scientist, UCLA Center for Health Services and Society, Los Angeles, California

CHRISTINA MANGURIAN, MD, MAS
Professor and Vice Chair for Diversity and Health Equity, UCSF Department of Psychiatry, San Francisco, California

MYRA L. MATHIS, MD
Attending Psychiatrist, Strong Recovery and Senior Instructor, Department of Psychiatry, University of Rochester, Rochester, New York

BRIAN McGREGOR, PhD
Associate Director of Research, Kennedy Satcher Center for Mental Health Equity, Satcher Health Leadership Institute, Assistant Professor of Psychiatry, Morehouse School of Medicine, Atlanta, Georgia

CHIRLANE I. McCRAY, ScD (Hon)
First Lady of New York City, New York, New York

STEVEN LEIFMAN, JD
Associative Administrative Judge, Miami-Dade County Court Eleventh Judicial Circuit of Florida, Miami, Florida

COURTNEY L. McMICKENS, MD, MPH, MHS
Forensic Mental Health Consultant, Lorio Forensics, Atlanta, Georgia

JEANNE MIRANDA, PhD
Professor, Department of Psychiatry and Biobehavioral Sciences, University of California, Los Angeles, Assistant Director, UCLA's Center for Health Services and Society, Los Angeles, California

QUIANTA MOORE, MD, JD
Fellow in Child Health Policy, Center for Health and Biosciences, Rice University's Baker Institute for Public Policy, Houston, Texas

LAUREN M. NUTILE, MD, MS
Child Psychiatry Fellow, Virginia Treatment Center for Children, Virginia Commonwealth University Health System, Richmond, Virginia

TEMI OLAFUNMILOYE
Research Assistant, The Disparities Solutions Center, Massachusetts General Hospital, Boston, Massachusetts

ROBERT M. ROHRBAUGH, MD
Professor of Psychiatry, Deputy Chair for Education and Career Development, Residency Program Director, Associate Dean for Global Health Education, Yale School of Medicine, New Haven, Connecticut

STEVEN M. STARKS, MD
Clinical Assistant Professor, Department of Clinical Sciences, University of Houston College of Medicine, Houston, Texas

DONNA M. SUDAK, MD
Professor of Psychiatry, Vice Chair for Education, Program Director, Drexel-Tower Health Psychiatry, Drexel University, Philadelphia, Pennsylvania

ANDRIA TATEM, MD
Instructor, Department of Pediatrics, Baylor College of Medicine, Texas Children's Hospital, Houston, Texas

PATRICK S. TENNANT, PhD, MS
Project Manager in Child Health Policy, Center for Health and Biosciences, Rice University's Baker Institute for Public Policy, Houston, Texas

NHI-HA TRINH, MD, MPH
Director, Massachusetts General Hospital (MGH), Department of Psychiatry Center for Diversity, Director of Multicultural Studies, Director of Clinical Services, MGH Depression Clinical and Research Program (DCRP), Assistant Professor of Psychiatry, Harvard Medical School (HMS), Associate Director of Holmes Society, HMS MGH DCRP, Boston, Massachusetts

SADE C. UDOETUK, MD
Assistant Professor, Menninger Department of Psychiatry and Behavioral Sciences, Baylor College of Medicine, Houston, Texas

JÜRGEN UNÜTZER, MD, MPH, MA
Professor and Chair, Department of Psychiatry and Behavioral Sciences, University of Washington, Seattle, Washington

SARAH Y. VINSON, MD
Associate Professor of Psychiatry and Pediatrics, Morehouse School of Medicine, Principal Consultant, Lorio Forensics, Atlanta, Georgia

SALA WEBB, MD, CPH, FAPA, DFAACAP
Chief Medical Officer, Behavioral Health, Comprehensive Medical and Dental Plan, Arizona Department of Child Safety, Phoenix, Arizona

KENNETH B. WELLS, MD, MPH
David Weil Endowed Chair and Professor, Department of Psychiatry and Biobehavioral Sciences, David Geffen School of Medicine, Department of Health Policy and Management, Fielding School of Public Health, Director, Center for Health Services and Society, UCLA Jane & Terry Semel Institute for Neuroscience & Human Behavior, Co-Director, California Center for Excellence in Behavioral Health, Staff Psychiatrist, Greater Los Angeles VA Health System, Los Angeles, California

Contents

> Significant mental health disparities persist in screening, diagnosis and
> treatment for racial and ethnic minorities compared with non-Latinx
> whites. Reducing mental health disparities, and ultimately achieving
> mental health equity, requires understanding the wide range of factors
> that influence health outcomes at multiple levels. Components of an effec-
> tive strategy to achieve mental health equity include increasing population-
> based care, increasing community-based health care services, addressing
> the social determinants of health, engaging the community, enhancing the
> pipeline and supporting a diverse, structurally competent workforce.

> More than 47 million Americans experience mental illness each year,
> and more than 9.2 million suffer from mental health and substance
> use disorders. More than 60% of adults with mental illness and 81%
> of those with substance use disorders do not receive treatment. As
> the human and financial costs from our nation's mental health and sub-
> stance use disorders crisis escalate, a strong business case to better
> address this crisis has emerged. This article describes the root causes
> and cost of disparities and offers an innovative perspective on aligning
> stakeholders to make the business case for equity in treatment and
> outcomes.

> This article offers a brief history of mental health policies that have
> shaped current inequities in health care financing and service delivery.
> Mental health has a unique position within the health care system
> given the pervasive nature of stigma associated with illness; race and
> ethnicity often amplify this burden. The acknowledgment of
> disparities in mental health and the development of policies that
> address the needs of minority groups are relatively recent phenomena.
> Highlighted are legislative actions that have influenced reforms of the
> health care landscape. This text outlines opportunities to advance a tar-
> geted, community-based approach to mental health policy
> development.

Racism is an important determinant of health and health disparities, but few strategies have been successful in eliminating racial discrimination from medical practice. This article proposes a novel antiracist approach to clinical care that acknowledges the racism shaping the clinical encounter and historical arc of racial oppression embedded in health care. Although preliminary, this approach can be easily implemented into clinical care and may reduce the harm done by racism. It could also serve as a template for antiracist service provision in other sectors, such as education and law enforcement.

This article briefly reviews the influences of protective and risk factors of child and adolescent mental health, and explores promising practices and outcomes of evidence-based programs designed to improve the mental health of youth, and the barriers for accessing quality and evidence-based child and adolescent mental health service delivery systems. The authors provide recommendations for individual practice improvements and policy, funding, and organizational practice improvements that will support mental health equity in child and adolescent populations.

Despite available treatment options for addiction, there remains an abysmal uptake of treatment initiation and engagement among varying communities. The existing treatment gap is based on historical occurrences, including discriminatory drug policies that have targeted communities of color with addiction. The current opioid epidemic and differential treatment therein exemplifies the severity of the existing disparity in addiction treatment, highlighting barriers such as institutionalized racism and vulnerabilities in the social determinants of health. To mitigate the disparity, an array of solutions to address these inequities are discussed, thereby providing a pathway forward to eliminating this treatment gap.

The literature supports the effectiveness of systems-based integrated care models, particularly collaborative care, to improve access, quality of care, and health outcomes for behavioral health conditions. There is growing evidence for the promise of collaborative care to reduce behavioral health disparities for racial and ethnic, low-income, and other at-risk populations. Using rapid literature review, this article highlights what is known about how collaborative care may promote health equity for behavioral health conditions, by reducing disparities in access, quality, and outcomes of care. Further, it explores innovative intervention and engagement strategies to promote behavioral health equity for at-risk groups.

There are historical predicates for the inequities noted in present-day community mental health. Stigma has led to discrimination for those living with mental illness. It is more difficult for research to occur, and to access care (prevention, early identification, evidence-based treatment services) because funding is limited and workforce development curtailed. Strategies to decrease stigma are suggested, means to enhance funding are offered, and models for workforce development are noted. Different treatment delivery systems are suggested to recruit and retain sufficient numbers of culturally competent and trauma-informed providers, so as to maximize access to necessary services.

The mental health system is often not readily accessible, culturally responsive, or a reliable source of effective interventions for society's most vulnerable populations. Modern-era studies estimate the number of persons diagnosed with serious mental illness in correctional facilities is more than 3 times the amount in hospitals. Understanding mass incarceration and the criminalization of mental illness is imperative to address mental health inequities. This article examines the interplay of mental health and criminal justice inequities, the historical context for the prevailing extant approaches to correctional mental health treatment, and programmatic approaches to addressing these inequities.

Severe mental health inequities exist in the United States, with reduced access to community-based care and poorer recovery outcomes associated with people of color, women, and lesbian, gay, bisexual, or transgender individuals. One strategy to reduce this inequity is to incorporate the perspectives of mental health consumers and their families into care planning and delivery. Successful integration of personal experience with evidence-based interventions can help reduce stigma and improve retention in care. To leverage public policy to reduce mental health inequity, New York City has launched ThriveNYC, the nation's largest municipal-level investment in mental health.

This article highlights the history of the psychiatric training practices that have contributed to inequity in mental health service delivery, particularly

PSYCHIATRIC CLINICS OF NORTH AMERICA

SERIES OF RELATED INTEREST

Child and Adolescent Psychiatric Clinics of North America
https://www.childpsych.theclinics.com/

Neurologic Clinics
https://www.neurologic.theclinics.com/

THE CLINICS ARE AVAILABLE ONLINE!
Access your subscription at:
www.theclinics.com

Preface

Achieving Mental Health Equity

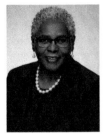   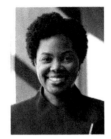

Altha J. Stewart, MD   Ruth S. Shim, MD, MPH
Editors

Developing an equitable mental health system has been a dream since my residency in the early 1980s. Throughout my career leading large urban mental health systems, I recognized that health disparities limited treatment options based on race and ethnicity. Leading up to my 2018 American Psychiatric Association (APA) presidency, it became clear that achieving the goal of mental health equity would require specific actions at a national level by leaders who made it a priority. It was for that reason I chose to include diversity and inclusion in my presidential agenda as part of a strategy to reduce the disparities in health and mental health that negatively impact the psychological health of underserved populations, especially racial and ethnic minorities. Throughout my presidency, I spoke of the APA's inconsistent history in creating strategies for eliminating mental health disparities and inequities. Although some progress was made, I also realized that such a laudable goal would not be achieved by 1 president over a 1-year term, so I partnered with Dr Ruth Shim on this special issue of *Psychiatric Clinics* to create a North Star to keep us focused on the ongoing work required to truly achieve mental health equity.

The recent murders of George Floyd, Breonna Taylor, and Ahmaud Arbery, coupled with the current coronavirus disease (COVID-19) pandemic has exposed the world to something that many of us have understood for a long time, that health problems differentially affect different populations, and that those populations that are more often marginalized or oppressed have worse outcomes than other populations. And yet, throughout this increased focus on disparities and inequities, much confusion persists about what causes these differences in outcomes. Are they, as the US Surgeon General Dr Jerome Adams implied, the result of poor choices by individuals? Or do health inequities exist because of unequal and unjust policies and practices?

This special issue explores the root causes of mental health inequities across a wide range of topics and considerations and focuses on solutions for achieving mental health equity. The articles in this issue build on each other to help unpack what has

Psychiatr Clin N Am 43 (2020) xiii–xiv
https://doi.org/10.1016/j.psc.2020.06.004
0193-953X/20/© 2020 Published by Elsevier Inc.

psych.theclinics.com

historically been misunderstood: the true drivers of mental health inequities. Initial articles help to frame the overall issue of mental health equity and discuss financial and policy considerations. We explore mental health equity from the clinical perspective, and focus on distinct populations and care delivery settings, including child and adolescent psychiatry, addictions, collaborative care, community psychiatry, and the criminal justice system. We will consider the consumer/family, training/education, and research perspectives in achieving mental health equity.

There is much work to be done to address mental health inequities and to begin to close the gaps that we see in mental health care and outcomes for many populations. James Baldwin once said, "Ignorance, allied with power, is the most ferocious enemy justice can have." This issue aims to reduce ignorance as it relates to mental health inequity, and to inspire us all to mobilize to begin to use our collective power to make a difference.

Altha J. Stewart, MD
The University of Tennessee
Health Science Center
920 Madison Avenue
Memphis, TN 38163, USA

Ruth S. Shim, MD, MPH
University of California, Davis
2230 Stockton Boulevard
Sacramento, CA 95817, USA

E-mail addresses:
astewa59@uthsc.edu (A.J. Stewart)
rshim@ucdavis.edu (R.S. Shim)

Mental Health Equity in the Twenty-First Century

Setting the Stage

Jean-Marie Alves-Bradford, MD[a],*, Nhi-Ha Trinh, MD, MPH[b],
Eraka Bath, MD[c,d,e], Angela Coombs, MD[f,g,1],
Christina Mangurian, MD, MAS[h]

KEYWORDS

- Equity • Disparities • Race • Ethnicity • Interventions

KEY POINTS

- Racial and ethnic disparities in mental health screening, diagnosis, and treatment are persistent barriers to mental health equity.
- Multilevel interventions are required to achieve mental health equity.
- Health care system reform to increase access and incentivize population-based care is critical to achieve mental health equity.
- Engaging community-based organizations, and developing the pipeline and workforce are key strategies to achieve mental health equity.
- Training at multiple levels (providers, patients, and communities) is needed to eliminate bias and stigma and create structural competence.

INTRODUCTION

Health care disparities are defined as differences in health care services received by two groups that are not caused by differences in underlying health care needs or preferences of group members but by the structure of the health care system, provider or patient biases, or clinical uncertainty.[1] The groundbreaking Surgeon General's report,

[a] New York State Psychiatric Institute, Washington Heights Community Service, Columbia University Department of Psychiatry, 1051 Riverside Drive, Box 112, New York, NY 10032, USA; [b] Department of Psychiatry Center for Diversity, MGH Depression Clinical and Research Program (DCRP), Harvard Medical School (HMS), HMS, Massachusetts General Hospital (MGH), One Bowdoin Square, 6th Floor, Boston, MA 02114-2790, USA; [c] Child Forensic Services; [d] Jane and Terry Semel Institute for Neuroscience and Human Behavior at UCLA; [e] Department of Psychiatry, 760 Westwood Plaza, Room A8-228 Los Angeles, CA 90024, USA; [f] Columbia University Department of Psychiatry; [g] Washington Heights Community Service, New York State Psychiatric Institute; [h] UCSF Department of Psychiatry, 1001 Potrero Avenue, Room 7M20, UCSF Box 0852, San Francisco, CA 94110, USA
[1] Present address: 1051 Riverside Drive, Box 112, New York, NY 10032.
* Corresponding author.
E-mail address: ja658@cumc.columbia.edu

Psychiatr Clin N Am 43 (2020) 415–428
https://doi.org/10.1016/j.psc.2020.05.001
0193-953X/20/© 2020 Elsevier Inc. All rights reserved.

Mental Health: Culture, Race, and Ethnicity in 2001 found that racial and ethnic minorities are less likely to receive needed care; when they do receive care, it is often lacking in quality compared with their white counterparts.[2] Significant disparities persist in the diagnosis and treatment of mental health issues for racial and ethnic minorities compared with non-Latinx white people (referred to as white people for the remainder of the article).[3]

Social-Ecological Model

Social determinants of health (SDOH) are the circumstances in which people are born, live, and work, as well as the systems put in place to support health care.[4] Taking this view, mental health disparities are the end result of larger social, economic, environmental, and structural inequities affecting marginalized communities.[4] Reducing mental health disparities, and achieving mental health equity, requires a broader social-ecological model approach, moving beyond individual behavior and toward an understanding of a range of mechanisms that influence health outcomes at multiple levels: individual, interpersonal, organizational/institutional, community, and policy.[4,5] For the individual level, mechanisms are patients' and providers' mental health and health system knowledge, attitudes, beliefs, and skills as well as communication barriers, which can be influenced by patient and provider biases or cultural differences.[6] At the interpersonal level, mechanisms are families, friends, and social networks. At the institutional level, mechanisms are organizations and social institutions. At the community level, mechanisms are relationships among organizations. At the systemic level, the mechanisms are national, state, and local policies, laws, and regulations.[5] Systemic factors include laws regarding insurance coverage that may lead to patients inability to access health care as a result of being uninsured or underinsured. Rather than working independently, these barriers may intersect, leading to racial and ethnic minorities receiving unequal mental health care.

COMPONENTS OF AN EFFECTIVE STRATEGY TO ACHIEVE MENTAL HEALTH EQUITY

Developing an effective strategy to achieve mental health equity involves interventions at multiple social-ecological levels (**Table 1**).

SYSTEMS INTERVENTIONS

Payment and delivery system models that incorporate improvement in value and quality outcomes are critical factors in achieving mental health equity.

Payment Reform

Federal and state systems-level change in payment and delivery models are needed to incentivize population-based care, a key element in achieving mental health equity. Current fee-for-service models reward volume regardless of the quality of services. As health systems move toward reimbursing bundled episodes of care, they will be more likely to incorporate changes in their systems that improve the overall health of individuals. Mental disorders are the costliest and most burdensome conditions in the United States and will need to be better integrated into health system reform.[7] The Affordable Care Act (ACA) has improved insurance coverage and use, especially in disadvantaged groups (black people, Latinx, and the poor), but disparities in care in these groups persist.[8] Fourteen states have currently opted out of the ACA Medicaid expansion, and Medicaid payments remain lower than private insurance, resulting in many health systems creating separate and unequal clinical services for Medicaid

Table 1
Components of an effective strategy to achieve mental health equity

Intervention	Examples
Systems Interventions	
Payment Reform	• Incentivize Population based care • Link Payment to outcomes • Bundle episodes of care
Delivery System Reform	• Increase Access to Mental Health Care • Increase Integrated Care Settings and Training • Increase Crisis and Community Based Services • Address Social Determinants of Health (housing, food insecurity, employment, transportation)
Community and Institutional Interventions	
Engage Community Based Organizations	• Mental Health Awareness and Anti-stigma campaigns for community and police
Form Community Coalitions	• Ex Crisis Intervention Teams
Improve Cultural and Linguistic Services	• Increase linguistic and cultural interpreters
Pipeline Development	• Recruitment and anti-stigma campaigns focusing on schools in workforce shortage settings
Workforce Development	• Mentorship, sponsorship, competitive salaries
Individual and Interpersonal Interventions	
Provider Education	• Improve patient-therapist communication • Bias Reduction training • Structural competence training • Use Structured Tools: diagnostic instruments, cultural formulations, medication algorithms
Patient Education	• Health Literacy Education • Anti-Stigma interventions • Patient activation and empowerment

recipients. Large-scale, organized efforts are needed for change. One such example, the federal Delivery System Reform Incentive Payment (DSRIP) program, has shown improved quality outcomes. DSRIP reformed the Medicaid system by requiring health care entities to partner with local community agencies and making payments contingent on outcomes such as decreasing avoidable hospitalizations.[9]

Delivery System Reform

Improve access
Closing the profound gap between treatment need and treatment receipt for racial and ethnic minority populations is essential to reach health equity.[10] Underrepresented racial and ethnic groups underuse mental health services compared with white people.[11] Structural barriers, including availability and proximity of appropriate facilities in a geographic location and limited mental health referrals, affect marginalized populations' ability to access quality mental health care.[12] Stockdale and colleagues[13] found that both black and Latinx populations were less likely to receive referrals for

counseling in both primary care and psychiatric settings compared with white populations. This finding is significant, particularly in primary care settings, because underrepresented racial and ethnic groups are more likely to seek mental health treatment from their primary care physicians than other settings.[14] When racial and ethnic minorities do access care, they are less likely to continue psychiatric treatment. In a nationally representative sample of racial and ethnic minorities, black people and Asian Americans with a history of depression within the past 12 months were less likely than white people to remain in treatment despite the need to continue.[15] Fortuna and colleagues[15] found that when black, Latinx, and Asian American patients were seen by a mental health specialist (vs a primary care provider) and were prescribed medication (vs therapy alone), they were significantly more likely to remain in treatment. Having a mental health specialist (vs a primary care provider) resulted in the greatest impact on treatment retention.

Increase integrated care settings and training opportunities

People with mental illness die 10 to 25 years earlier than the general population because of medical illnesses similar to the leading causes of death nationwide.[16] Practices that effectively integrate behavioral and primary care have been shown to improve clinical outcomes, satisfaction, wellness, and quality of life for patients and health system cost savings.[17] Professional organizations identify the need for increased training in integrated care settings to prepare providers to address the health of people with mental illness.[18] Integrated care training opportunities are increasing in US residencies and through integrated care fellowships. Innovative programs, such as the Satcher Health Leadership Institute at the Morehouse School of Medicine, develop leaders who will help to promote health equity by providing clinical and administrative health care professionals with knowledge and training to develop culturally sensitive integrated care practices.[17]

Increase crisis and community services

Shifting care from high-cost inpatient and hospital-based emergency services to community-based locations providing crisis services, care coordination, and increased community support will decrease cost and increase improvement in outcomes and patient satisfaction. Peer providers, patient navigators, and community health workers have been shown to foster hope, trust, and empowerment in the communities they serve and to increase access and quality through care coordination.[19]

Address social determinants of health

As health systems bear more of the risk and cost for care, they take on the responsibility of improving the SDOH in order to improve health care conditions. The American Medical Association (AMA) and an insurer, United Healthcare, recently created International Classification of Diseases-10 (ICD-10) codes related to the SDOH, which provide a standard way for health systems to monitor SDOH.[20] Several insurers and hospital systems have invested financial resources to provide housing and health care on site at housing locations to decrease costly inpatient and emergency use.[21] Insurers are covering transportation services to medical appointments and some hospitals and medical providers are partnering with ride-share services to increase access to services. Integrated SDOH-targeted interventions such as individualized placement and support, which helps individuals obtain employment services, result in reductions in hospitalizations and improvements in social functioning.[22]

INSTITUTIONAL AND COMMUNITY INTERVENTIONS
Partner with Community-Based Programs

Partnering with community-based programs and key sociocultural institutions within vulnerable communities is critically important in achieving mental health equity. One example of a mental health intervention that can work synergistically within trusted institutions and community sites (eg, faith-based organizations, schools, beauty salons, barbershops) is Mental Health First Aid (MHFA). MHFA is a skills-based course that trains participants to identify signs of a mental health or substance use crisis and assist others to obtain help.[23] Originally developed in Australia, it is a widely disseminated evidence-based program that shows improvement in knowledge of mental health problems and treatments, changes in attitudes toward mental illness, and increases in self-reported helping behaviors.[23,24] By offering MHFA trainings in community sites such as churches, mosques, schools, and barbershops, members of traditionally underserved communities are empowered with tools to both identify signs of mental health crises and connect others to important mental health resources. This program simultaneously supports reducing levels of stigma and increasing help-seeking for a mental health concern.

Form Community Coalitions

Forming community coalitions lays a foundation for meaningful and impactful community engagement and change. Coalitions are commonly composed of community members, key stakeholders, and individuals from institutions (eg, academic, hospitals, government agencies) that can provide resources or technical assistance.[25] In addressing the specific needs and vulnerabilities of the community from which coalition members are connected, coalitions decrease the odds of alienating community members with the initiatives developed. By creating culturally appropriate and in-tune interventions, community coalitions can increase the odds of sustaining meaningful change. In a 10-year follow-up study examining the impact of a community coalition formed in one of the poorest neighborhoods in Kansas City, Missouri, researchers found that the coalition was effective in implementing 117 community changes that were associated with improvements in SDOH, specifically housing and crime reduction, and most of the changes were sustained over a decade.[26]

Crisis intervention teams (CITs) are an example of coalitions helping to address mental health disparities. Nationwide, CITs bring together law enforcement, mental health professionals, consumers, and their advocates to develop and implement strategies to divert individuals living with mental illness from the criminal justice system, where they are disproportionately represented.[27] Research has shown lower self-perceived use of force among officers and diversion from prebooking in jails to psychiatric facilities.[28]

A novel model for improving the health of a community is the University of California, San Francisco (UCSF) Anchor Institution Initiative.[29] Anchor institutions are place-based, mission-driven entities (such as hospitals, universities, and government agencies) that leverage their economic power alongside their human and intellectual resources to improve the long-term health and social welfare of their communities. Through this initiative, UCSF is exploring social impact investment options; supporting local businesses that employ under-resourced populations; and increasing its capacity to train, hire, and promote people from under-resourced populations.

Culturally and Linguistically Appropriate Services

Limited English proficiency is closely associated with the underuse of psychiatric services and a longer duration of untreated illness.[30] In a study of white, black, Asian, and

Latinx populations, among subjects who spoke no English and specified a need for mental health care, only 8% of them received such care, versus 51% of subjects who spoke English only, and 42% of subjects who were bilingual.[31] In 2001, the US Department of Health and Human Services issued national guidelines on Culturally Linguistically Appropriate Services (CLAS) Standards for clinicians, organizations, and state agencies. The National CLAS Standards emphasize the importance of communication and language assistance to facilitate access for individuals with limited English proficiency and/or communication needs and to recruit a culturally and linguistically diverse workforce.[32] A recent review revealed that most states have not fully adopted these standards, nor are agencies receiving federal assistance providing language services to the standards set by the Office of Mental Health.[33,34] Establishing institutional policies that require collecting data on patients' preferred languages and establishing a reliable and effective process by which patients can gain access to interpreter services is crucial. In addition to language fluency, cultural fluency is important as well. Many patients prefer mental health providers of the same ethnicity, perceive therapists of the same ethnicity more positively, and some ethnic groups show improvement in outcomes when the provider and the patient are of the same racial or ethnic background.[35]

Pipeline Development

Lack of diversity within the physician-scientist workforce is a barrier to achieving mental health equity operating at multiple levels, including individual, interpersonal, community, and institutional. The Association of American Medical Colleges (AAMC) defines underrepresented in medicine (URM) as those racial and ethnic populations that are underrepresented in the medical profession relative to their numbers in the general population.[36] Only 5.8% of physicians identify as Latinx, whereas Latinx people are 18% of the US population; 5% of physicians identify as black, whereas black people are 14% of the US population; and Native American physicians are less than 0.5% and are 0.9% of the US population.[36,37] Studies show that physicians from underrepresented groups are more likely to work in underserved areas and engage in research related to health disparities and underserved populations.[38] The authors propose that the best approach to diversify the mental health workforce is an anti-stigma and recruitment campaign throughout the education system, starting in elementary school and continuing through residency.

Elementary and middle school

Systems leaders should promote anti-stigma campaigns as early as elementary school. Although mental health is increasingly recognized as being a critical component of well-being and is being promoted at all levels of education in resource-rich settings, anti-stigma campaigns should focus on schools in mental health workforce shortage settings, which often have a high proportion of URM students. Anti-stigma campaigns will not only help with early identification but also may inspire youth to pursue careers in mental health.

High school

Early high school is an ideal age to be exposed to strong leaders in mental health because role modeling is crucial. The American Psychiatric Association (APA) Doctors Back to School program is modeled after the AMA's Doctors Back to School Program.[39] It sends URM physicians and medical students into the community to introduce children to professional role models and shows children of all ages from URM groups that a career in medicine is attainable for everyone. The successful UCSF

High School Intern program matches urban public-school students who are not yet on the path to college with a UCSF scientist mentor.[40] Most of these students are from backgrounds underrepresented in science.

College
Outreach should be targeted to recruit URM students at historically black colleges and universities and Hispanic-serving institutions. To address declining URM medical school applicants, the APA created 3 workforce inclusion pipeline programs, 1 for black male students, 1 for Native American students, and 1 for Latinx students. The APA Black Men in Psychiatry Early Pipeline Program recruits undergraduate Howard University students interested in medicine.[41] It provides exposure to psychiatry, community activities, financial support for Medical College Admission Test preparation, and mentoring. Medical education research shows that a diverse training environment has cross-sectional advantages where all students benefit from increased cognitive complexity, civic-mindedness, and increased knowledge and understanding of other cultures and experiences.[38]

Medical school
URM medical students should be actively recruited and supported to choose psychiatry. Medical schools should encourage participation in several of the national psychiatry medical student programs, such as travel scholarships, fellowships, and early pipeline programs to increase exposure to psychiatry. Several calls to action have been made by national science and educational organizations to prioritize the diversification of the biomedical and scientific workforce. These efforts include those by the National Institutes of Health (NIH), the National Academy of Sciences, the American Committee on Graduate Medical Education (ACGME), and the AAMC. Beginning July 2019, the ACGME implemented standards around equity, diversity, and inclusion to engage in systematic, intentional, and structural efforts to increase retention and recruitment of those who are underrepresented from students to faculty, administration, and staff. Similarly, the AAMC's advancement of holistic review initiatives has broadened the lens by which applications are considered. Holistic reviews allow admissions committees to consider a broad range of factors, including experiences and attributes in addition to academic performance.[42]

Residency
There are several APA fellowships that all psychiatry residents are eligible for. Departments of Psychiatry should operationalize sponsorship of residents from underrepresented backgrounds to participate in these fellowships. One of these fellowships, the Substance Abuse and Mental Health Services Administration Minority Fellowship, is particularly notable because it is associated with significant funds for the individual awardee.[43] These fellowships not only advance the careers of URM residents but also help with leadership training and connect fellows with peer and senior mentorship.

Workforce Development
There is a clear need not only to strengthen the pipeline but also for institutions to support those who are working in public psychiatry settings. Work in the public sector can be challenging given the high prevalence of trauma and the impact of structural racism, which can often seem outside of the capacity to treat. As such, these providers are at risk of burnout. URM providers who experience microaggressions and macroaggressions at work may be even more at risk in certain settings. There are several solutions to help strengthen the supports for a diverse workforce, including mentorship, sponsorship, and funding.

Mentorship and sponsorship

Mentorship is critical for all employees. Junior employees should be paired with senior mentors, ideally in some leadership roles for role modeling. If resources are limited, peer networks should be established and referral to national mentoring programs should be operationalized. Although mentors give advice and feedback, sponsors are in positions of power and use their influence to create opportunities for others. Leaders should intentionally sponsor employees from under-represented backgrounds for national awards and/or mentoring opportunities (eg, the AAMC Early Career Women Faculty Leadership Development Seminar).[44] Similarly, these individuals should be nominated for leadership positions that are associated with protected time, salary, and control of funds.

Funding

Salaries for working in public settings should be commensurate with private settings. Leadership should actively encourage participation in loan repayment programs and provide support to help candidates prepare these applications. In academic settings, URM women tend to have a high proportion of women and URM mentees. These so-called supermentors bear a minority tax, a burden of extra unreimbursed responsibilities placed on URM faculty in the name of diversity.[45] These mentoring roles should be reimbursed with protected time and additional salary support, because this will benefit the next generation of women and URM in the health workforce, who need to be protected from burnout from this unreimbursed work.

PROVIDER INTERVENTIONS
Provider Education on Bias and Reducing Disparities

Racial and ethnic diagnostic disparities within psychiatry is a persistent problem and has implications across the continuum from assessment to diagnosis to intervention. Black and Latinx patients are 3 times more likely to receive a psychotic disorder diagnosis compared with white patients.[46] Black patients are less likely to receive a diagnosis of an affective disorder, and black patients with bipolar disorder have significantly higher rates of receiving an initial clinical diagnosis other than bipolar disorder, which can delay treatment that can directly affect morbidity.[47,48] Implicit biases influence health decision making at various points, with adverse health outcomes and increased morbidity and mortality for nonwhite patients.[49] Hoffman and colleagues[49] found that approximately 50% of medical students and residents surveyed thought that black patients feel less pain compared with white patients based on false beliefs (eg, hat black people's skin is thicker than white people's skin) and, as a result, were more likely to suggest inappropriate treatments for black patients compared with white patients. Alegría and colleagues[50] found that, compared with white people, racial and ethnic minorities received less standard depression care, defined as receiving either (1) antidepressant use for the past month combined with 4 or more treatment visits in the past year, or (2) 8 or more treatment visits of at least 30 minutes' duration, without antidepressant use, in the past year. Racial and ethnic minorities are less likely to receive antidepressants for depression diagnoses compared with white people.[51] Latinx populations are much less likely to receive comparable treatment of pain, and a Latinx man is 50% less likely to receive opioids for a broken leg and 7 times less likely to receive opioids than a white man in an emergency room even when physicians assessed the pain accurately.[52,53] Treatment disparities in psychotic disorders include increased doses of antipsychotics, increased restraints, and decreased clozapine use in black people compared with white people.[54,55] Black, Latinx, and Asian Americans are all less likely to receive equivalent mental health care compared with white people, including physicians spending less time with and delivering less information to racial and ethnic minorities.[50,51,56] Implicit bias research shows that providers who score higher on the Implicit Association Test are less likely to provide equal treatment to black and Latinx patients who present with similar symptoms to white people.[57] Disrupting bias is thus critical to achieving equity. Providers should be aware of and try to modify their own biases and microaggressions in the clinical encounter.[58]

Training in Structural Competency

Providers should be given training in structural competence so that they have tools to address challenges facing their patients and families. Structural competency is the ability to discern how systems and the SDOH affect clinical interaction.[59] Structural barriers lead to structural vulnerability in racial and ethnic minority populations, defined as "an individual's or a population group's condition of being at risk for negative health outcomes through their interface with socioeconomic, political, and cultural/normative hierarchies."[12] Providers should consider the ability of patients to follow recommended treatment regimens in their environments and make suggestions on how to achieve treatment goals in their context.

Use Standardized Tools

Using standardized tools such as diagnostic instruments, cultural formulations, and medication and treatment algorithms can reduce bias. Studies have shown significant changes to diagnosis with the use of semistructured instruments for diagnosis and strict adherence to criteria.[60] Training in the use of the Diagnostic and Statistical Manual of Mental Disorders, Fifth Edition (DSM-5) Cultural Formulation Interview improves providers' cultural competence, and using medication algorithms has been shown to decrease disparities.[61,62]

Improve Communication

Improving patient-therapist communication can improve outcomes such as treatment initiation, participation, and continuation.[53] Providers should avoid assumptions and should use interview techniques such as asking open-ended questions to understand the patient's context and symptoms. Providers should be aware of historical context, cultural mistrust, and the role of stigma. Patients often feel disempowered in medical settings and can experience feeling not heard or not having their values represented, especially in times when treatments are not effective. Provider interventions such as using shared decision making, speaking with jargon-free language, tailoring communication and treatment plans to patient preferences, discussing clinician backgrounds, acknowledging power differentials, and observing differences in communication styles may improve participation in treatment.[63,64]

PATIENT INTERVENTIONS

At the core of the social-ecological model lies the intrapersonal level where interventions can specifically target patients' mental health knowledge and beliefs about mental illness, including internalized stigma and skillfulness in navigating a complex mental health landscape. In addition to increasing patients' basic mental health literacy, there is also a need to equip patients with the knowledge of which services they may benefit from and their rights in clinical encounters. For example, patients may be unaware of parity laws that require insurance plans to provide mental health and substance use services that are not more restrictive than their medical coverage. Patients may similarly be unaware of their right to appeal a denied claim.

Anti-stigma interventions are particularly important when addressing the unmet mental health needs of marginalized and minority communities because they often experience significantly higher levels of stigma.[65] Decreasing levels of internalized stigma are important because both stigma and illness identity can affect patients' courses of recovery.[66] Several anti-stigma interventions have shown promising results, including Ending Self-Stigma (ESS) and Anti-Stigma Photovoice.[67] ESS is a 9-session psychoeducation course for adults living with serious mental illness that uses a combination of reflection, teaching, skills, and home-based practice. One pilot study showed a significant decrease in internalized stigma and an increase in perceived recovery.[68] The Anti-Stigma PhotoVoice Program is a 10-week group in which participants receive psychoeducation about stigma and use photography as a tool to explore and share their own narratives and lived experiences with mental illness. The Anti-Stigma PhotoVoice Program showed a significant effect on both decreasing stigma and improving coping with stigma in a randomized control trial.[69]

Many factors contribute to lower levels of treatment retention and engagement among minority populations compared with white people. Minority patients often experience being less participatory in visits with providers, particularly if those providers are not from the same race.[70] Patient activation interventions such as The Right Question Project teaches and prepares patients to ask questions during appointments to obtain meaningful information from their providers. When studied in a majority Latinx, Spanish-speaking population, participants who received the intervention were more than twice as likely to engage and continue in treatment.[71]

SUMMARY

Significant disparities persist in the screening, diagnosis, and treatment of mental health issues for racial and ethnic minorities compared with white people. Reducing mental health disparities, and ultimately achieving mental health equity, requires understanding the wide range of factors that influence health outcomes at multiple social ecologic levels. Components of an effective strategy to achieve mental health equity include (1) increasing access with delivery and payment systems–level reform, incentivizing population-based care, and linking payments to outcomes; (2) working directly with communities and coalitions to improve services; (3) increasing the pipeline and diversifying the workforce; and (4) empowering patients with intrapersonal interventions and developing structural competence in providers.

DISCLOSURE

Dr J.M. Alves-Bradford has nothing to disclose.

REFERENCES

1. Smedley BD, Stith AY, Nelson AR, editors. Unequal treatment: confronting racial and ethnic disparities in health care. Washington, DC: National Academies Press (US); 2003.
2. U.S Department of Health and Human Services. Mental health: culture, race, and ethnicity-A supplement to mental health: a report of the Surgeon general. Rockville (MD): US Department of Health and Human Services, Substance Abuse and Mental Health Services Administration, Center for Mental Health Services; 2001.

3. Cook B, Trinh N, Li Z, et al. Trends in racial-ethnic disparities in access to mental health care, 2004-2012. Psychiatric Services; 2017. p. 68–9.
4. Sheiham A. Closing the gap in a generation: health equity through action on the social determinants of health. A report of the World Health Organization Commission on Social Determinants of Health; 2008.
5. McLeroy KR, Bibeau D, Steckler A, et al. An ecological perspective on health promotion programs. Health Educ Q 1988;15(4):351–77.
6. Betancourt JR, Green AR, Carrillo JE, et al. Defining cultural competence: a practical framework for addressing racial/ethnic disparities in health and health care. Public Health Rep 2003;118(4):293–302.
7. Roehrig C. Mental disorders top the list of the most costly conditions in the United States: $201 billion. Health Aff (Millwood) 2016;35(6):1130–5.
8. Gaffney A, McCormick D. The affordable care act: implications for health-care equity. Lancet 2017;389:144–52.
9. Pourat N. California Public Hospitals Improved quality of care under Medicaid waiver program. UCLA Health Policy Brief; 2017 ;PB2017-4:1-10.
10. Walker E, Cummings JR, Hockenberry JM, et al. Insurance status, use of mental health services, and unmet need for mental health care in the United States. Psychiatr Serv 2015;66(6):578–84.
11. Substance Abuse and Mental Health Services Administration. Racial/ethnic differences in mental health service use among adults. Rockwille, MD: Substance Abuse and Mental Health Services Administration; 2015. HHS Publication No. SMA-15-4906.
12. Bourgois P, Holmes SM, Sue K, et al. Structural vulnerability: operationalizing the concept to address health disparities in clinical care. Acad Med 2017;92(3): 299–307.
13. Stockdale SE, Lagomasino IT, Siddique J, et al. Racial and ethnic disparities in detection and treatment of depression and anxiety among psychiatric and primary health care visits, 1995-2005. Med Care 2008;46(7):668–77.
14. Goodell S. Health Policy Brief: Mental Health Parity. Health Aff (Millwood) 2014. Available at: https://www.healthaffairs.org/do/10.1377/hpb20140403.871424/full/.
15. Fortuna LR, Alegria M, Gao S. Retention in depression treatment among ethnic and racial minority groups in the United States. Depress Anxiety 2010;27(5): 485–94. https://doi.org/10.1002/da.20685.
16. Colton CW, Manderscheid RW. Congruencies in increased mortality rates, years of potential life lost, and causes of death among public mental health clients in eight states. Prevent Chronic Dis 2006;3(2):A42.
17. Satcher D, Rachel S. Promoting mental health equity: the role of integrated care. J Clin Psychol Med Settings 2017;24:182–6.
18. Druss BG, Chwastiak L, Kern J, et al. Psychiatry's role in improving the physical health of patients with serious mental illness: a report from the American Psychiatric Association. Psychiatr Serv 2018;69(3):254–6.
19. Natale-Pereira A, Enard K, Nevarez L, et al. The role of patient navigators in eliminating health disparities. Cancer 2011;(15):3543–53.
20. UnitedHealthcare and the AMA collaborate to understand and address social barriers preventing people's access to better health. Available at: https://newsroom.uhc.com/content/uhc/newsroom/news-releases/AMA-announcement.html. Accessed December 30, 2019.
21. Butcher L. "Why hospitals are housing the homeless" Hospitals and Health Networks 2017.

22. Burns T, Catty J, White S, et al. The impact of supported employment and working on clinical and social functioning: results of an international study of individual placement and support. Schizophr Bull 2009;35(5):949–58.
23. Wong EC, Collins RL, Cerully JL. Reviewing the evidence base for mental health first aid: is there support for its use with key target populations in California? Rand Health Q 2015;5(1):19.
24. Hadlaczky G, Hökby S, Mkrtchian A, et al. Mental Health First Aid is an effective public health intervention for improving knowledge, attitudes, and behaviour: A meta-analysis. Int Rev Psychiatry 2014;26:467–75.
25. Wolff T. Community coalition building—contemporary practice and research: introduction. Am J Community Psychol 2001;29(2):165–72.
26. Watson-Thompson J, May MJ, Jefferson J, et al. Examining the contributions of a community coalition in addressing urban health determinants. J Prev Interv Community 2018;46(1):7–27.
27. Watson AC, Fulambarker AJ. The crisis intervention team model of police response to mental health crises: a primer for mental health practitioners. Best Practices Ment Health 2012;8(2):71.
28. Rogers MS, McNiel DE, Binder RL. Effectiveness of Police Crisis Intervention Training Programs. J Am Acad Psychiatry Law 2019. https://doi.org/10.29158/JAAPL.003863-19.
29. University of California San Francisco Anchor Institution Initiative. Available at: https://anchor.ucsf.edu/. Accessed April 16, 2020.
30. Ohtani A, Suzuki T, Takeuchi H, et al. Language barriers and access to psychiatric care: a systematic review. Psychiatr Serv 2015;66(8):798–805.
31. Sentell T, Shumway M, Snowden L. Access to mental health treatment by english language proficiency and race/ethnicity. J Gen Intern Med 2007;22(2):289–93.
32. US Department of Health and Human Services: Office of Minority Health. National standards for culturally and linguistically appropriate services (CLAS) in health and health care. Rockville (MD): IQ Solutions Inc; 2001.
33. Aggarwal N, Cedeno K, John D, et al. Adoption of the National CLAS standards by state mental health agencies: A nationwide policy analysis. Psychiatr Serv 2017;68:856–8.
34. Green AR, Nze C. Language-Based Inequity in Health Care: Who Is the "Poor Historian?". AMA J Ethics 2017;19(3):263–71.
35. Cabral RR, Smith TB. Racial/Ethnic matching of clients and therapists in mental health services: A meta-analytic review of preferences, perceptions and outcomes. J Couns Psychol 2001;58(4):537–54.
36. AAMC Underrepresented in Medicine Definition. Available at: https://www.aamc.org/what-we-do/mission-areas/diversity-inclusion/underrepresented-in-medicine. Accessed December 29, 2019.
37. US census data.census.gov. Available at: https://data.census.gov/cedsci/table?q=Total Population in the United States. Accessed December 29, 2019.
38. Acosta D. Trends in Racial and Ethnic Minority Applicants and Matriculants to U.S. Medical Schools, 1980-2016. AAMC Analysis in Brief 2017;17:3.
39. American Medical Association's Doctors Back to School Program. Available at: https://www.ama-assn.org/member-groups-sections/minority-affairs/doctors-back-school-program. Accessed April 16, 2020.
40. University of California San Francisco High School Intern program. Available at: http://sep.ucsf.edu/hs_programs/high-school-intern-program. Accessed April 16, 2020.

41. APA Black Men in Psychiatry Early Pipeline Program. Available at: https://www.psychiatry.org/residents-medical-students/medical-students/medical-student-programs/workforce-inclusion-pipeline/black-men-in-psychiatry. Accessed April 16, 2020.

42. Holistic Review. Available at: https://www.aamc.org/services/member-capacity-building/holistic-review. Accessed April 3, 2020.

43. Substance Abuse and Mental Health Services Administration (SAMHSA) Minority Fellowship. Available at: https://www.psychiatry.org/residents-medical-students/residents/fellowships/available-apa-apaf-fellowships/samhsa-minority-fellowship. Accessed April 16, 2020.

44. AAMC Early Career Women Faculty Leadership Development Seminar). Available at: https://www.aamc.org/professional-development/leadership-development/ewims. Accessed April 16, 2020.

45. Rodríguez JE, Campbell KM, Pololi LH. Addressing disparities in academic medicine: what of the minority tax? BMC Med Educ 2015;15:6.

46. Schwartz R, Blankenship D. Racial disparities in psychotic disorder diagnosis: A review of empirical literature. Wold J Psyhciatry 2014;4(4):133–40.

47. Strakowski S, Keck PE Jr, Arnold LM, et al. Ethnicity and diagnosis in patients with affective disorders. J Clin Psychiatry 2003;64:7.

48. Akinhanmi MO, Biernacka JM, Strakowski SM, et al. Racial disparities in bipolar disorder treatment and research: a call to action. Bipolar Disord 2018;20(6):506–14.

49. Hoffman KM, Trawalter S, Axt JR, et al. Racial bias in pain assessment and treatment recommendations, and false beliefs about biological differences between blacks and whites. Proc Natl Acad Sci U S A 2016;113(16):4296–301.

50. Alegría M, Chatterji P, Wells K, et al. Disparity in depression treatment among racial and ethnic minority populations in the United States. Psychiatr Serv 2008;59(11):1264–72.

51. Simpson SM, Krishnan LL, Kunik ME, et al. Racial disparities in diagnosis and treatment of depression: a literature review. Psychiatr Q 2007;78(1):3–14.

52. Todd KH, Samaroo N, Hoffman JR. Ethnicity as a risk factor for inadequate emergency department analgesia. JAMA 1993;269(12):1537–9.

53. White IIIA, Chanoff D. Seeing patients unconscious bias in health care. Cambridge (MA): Harvard University Press; 2011.

54. Kelly DL, Dixon LB, Kreyenbuhl JA, et al. Clozapine utilization and outcomes by race in a public mental health system: 1994-2000. J Clin Psychiatry 2006;67(9):1404–11.

55. Diaz FJ, De Leon J. Excessive antipsychotic dosing in 2 U.S. State hospitals. J Clin Psychiatry 2002;63(11):998–1003.

56. Olfson M, Cherry DK, Lewis-Fernández R. Racial Differences in visit duration of outpatient psychiatric visits. Arch Gen Psychiatry 2009;66(2):214–21.

57. Fitzgerald C, Hurst S. Implicit bias in healthcare professionals: a systematic review. BMC Med Ethics 2017;18:19.

58. Sue D. Microaggressions in everyday life. Am Psychol 2007;62(4):271–86.

59. Metzl JM, Hansen H. Structural Competency: theorizing a new medical engagement with stigma and inequality. Soc Sci Med 2014;103:126–33.

60. Miller PR, Dasher R, Collins R, et al. Inpatient diagnostic assessments: 1. accuracy of structured vs unstructured interviews. Psychiatry Res 2001;105:255–64.

61. Aggarwal N, Lam P, Jiménez-Solomon O, et al. An online training module on the cultural formulation interview: the case of New York State. Psychiatr Serv 2018;69(11):1135–7.

62. Covell N, Jackson C, Evans AC, et al. Antipsychotic prescribing practices in Connecticut's public mental health system: rates of changing medications and prescribing styles. Schizophr Bull 2002;28(1):17–29.

63. Aggarwal N, Pieh M, Dixon L, et al. Clinician descriptions of communication strategies to improve treatment engagement by racial/ethnic minorities in mental health series: A systematic review. Patient Educ Couns 2016;99:198–209.

64. Elwyn G, Frosch D, Thomson R, et al. Shared decision making: a model for clinical practice. J Gen Intern Med 2012;27:1361–7.

65. Lee K. Understanding and addressing the stigma of mental illness with ethnic minority communities. Health Sociol Rev 2012;21(3):287–98.

66. Yanos PT, Roe D, Lysaker PH. The impact of illness identity on recovery from severe mental illness. Am J Psychiatr Rehabil 2010;13(2):73–93.

67. Yanos PT, Lucksted A, Drapalski AL, et al. Interventions targeting mental health self-stigma: A review and comparison. Psychiatr Rehabil J 2015;38(2):171.

68. Lucksted A, Drapalski A, Calmes C, et al. Ending self-stigma: Pilot evaluation of a new intervention to reduce internalized stigma among people with mental illnesses. Psychiatr Rehabil J 2011;35:51–4.

69. Russinova Z, Rogers ES, Gagne C, et al. A randomized controlled trial of a peer-run antistigma photovoice intervention. Psychiatr Serv 2014;65(2):242–6.

70. Cooper-Patrick L, Gallo J, Gonzales J, et al. Race, gender, and partnership in the patient-physician relationship. JAMA 1999;282:583–9.

71. Alegría M, Polo A, Gao S, et al. Evaluation of a patient activation and empowerment intervention in mental health care. Med Care 2008;46(3):247–56.

The Business Case for Mental Health Equity

James Corbett, MDiv, JD[a], Temi Olafunmiloye[b,1], Joseph R. Betancourt, MD, MPH[c,*]

KEYWORDS

• Mental health • Substance use disorder • Opioids • Disparities • Business case

KEY POINTS

• Racial and ethnic disparities persist in mental health and substance use disorders, as minorities face greater challenges accessing mental health and substance use disorder services and receive a lower quality of care.
• Mental health expenditure exceeds that of other medical conditions, increases the costs of addressing physical health, and is exacerbated by health disparities.
• Real-world evidence trials account for strategic and operational concerns along with the disparate financial incentives of multiple stakeholders.
• Real-world evidence trials offer great promise to solidify the business case for equity, reduce disparities, and combat the major challenge of mental health and substance use disorders.

INTRODUCTION

Mental health has garnered increased attention in recent years as more than 47 million Americans experience mental illness each year, and 9.2 million Americans suffer from mental health and substance use disorders (SUD).[1] The need for services to address this growing epidemic has become a public health and policy priority; more than 60% of adults with mental illness and 81% of those with SUD do not receive treatment.[1,2] Nevertheless, health system investment in mental health and SUD services remains challenging for multiple reasons, including low reimbursement and low return on investment as compared with more profitable health system services. At the same

[a] Initium Health, EO Health, 1401 Wewatta Street Suite 103, Denver, CO 80202, USA; [b] The Disparities Solutions Center, Massachusetts General Hospital, Boston, MA, USA; [c] Equity and Inclusion Administration, The Disparities Solutions Center, Massachusetts General Hospital, Harvard Medical School, 55 Fruit Street, Bulfinch Building, Room 127, Boston, MA 02114, USA
[1] Present address: 500 District Avenue, Burlington, MA 01803.
* Corresponding author.
E-mail address: jbetancourt@partners.org
Twitter: @JCETHICIST (J.C.); @Jbetancourtpr (J.R.B.)

Psychiatr Clin N Am 43 (2020) 429–438
https://doi.org/10.1016/j.psc.2020.04.001
0193-953X/20/© 2020 Elsevier Inc. All rights reserved.

Abbreviations	
MAT	Medications for addiction treatment
OUD	Opioid use disorder
SUD	Substance use disorders

time, payors historically have carved out mental health and SUD from physical health and reimbursed less for these services, and regulators have not appropriately monitored or enforced policies such as the Mental Health Parity and Addiction Equity Act. As the monetary and human costs from our nation's mental health and SUD burden escalate, however, strong business and ethical cases arise to better address this crisis in a meaningful and sustainable manner. This need is further magnified as our nation pushes toward value-based care and population health management, where improving outcomes and performance in physical health requires concomitant treatment of mental illness and SUD. This article describes the root causes and cost of disparities in mental health and SUD and offers an innovative perspective on aligning stakeholders to make the business case for equity in mental health and SUD treatment and outcomes.

A deeper exploration of the mental health and SUD crisis demonstrates that racial and ethnic disparities persist. For instance, minority populations tend to have limited access to health care, and receive lower quality care, than their white counterparts. Although research shows that minorities have a lower or equivalent prevalence of mental illnesses as whites, mental health services are more likely to be used by those that are white, high income, and living in urban areas.[3,4] Black and Latinx populations are less likely to receive mental health services and receive adequate quality care.[5–8] For example, between 2008 and 2012, whites had the highest average use of mental health services at 16.6%, followed by American Indian/Alaskan Natives (15.6%), African Americans (8.6%), Latinos (7.3%), and Asians (4.9%).[9] Further, the mental health needs of patients with limited English proficiency are dramatically unmet, with research revealing that only 8% of patients with limited English proficiency who express a need for services receive them.[10] Given that these minority and populations with limited English proficiency also disproportionately suffer from and receive lower quality care for chronic conditions such as heart disease, asthma, and diabetes, and because physical health outcomes worsen and costs increase by inadequate treatment of mental illness, an even stronger business case is evolving for mental health equity.

BACKGROUND ON MENTAL HEALTH AND SUBSTANCE USE DISORDERS
Disparities in Mental Health

Mental health disparities describe the unequal access to mental health services, lower quality of care, and decreased probability of favorable risk-adjusted health outcomes that minority groups experience.[11] Although mental health services use has generally increased in the United States over time, minority populations have faced greater challenges accessing them, for both historical and structural reasons. Mental health disparities are impacted by social and physical stressors that impact minority populations at greater rates.[12] These include racial discrimination and social exclusion; adverse early life experiences; poor education; unemployment, underemployment, and job insecurity; poverty, income inequality, and neighborhood deprivation; poor access to sufficient healthy food; poor housing quality and housing instability; adverse features of the built environment; and poor access to health care.[13] Generally, the greater the social inequality, the higher the risk of developing a mental health disorder.

Barriers to receiving mental health care are extensive. Research demonstrates that high cost and limited insurance coverage are the highest reported barriers to using mental health services among all racial and ethnic minority groups. Other barriers include stigma, negative experiences with providers, perceived ineffectiveness of treatment, and structural barriers such as limited appointment availability and lack of transportation.[14] For example, research has shown that black, Latinx, and Asian populations are more likely to report prejudice, discrimination, and a lack of confidence that the services would help as reasons for not seeking treatment.[9] The burden of mental health disparities is further exacerbated by the political climate. For example, 1 study showed that lesbian, gay, and bisexual populations living in states with bans on same-sex marriage had higher rates of psychological distress as compared with lesbian, gay, and bisexual populations living in states without these bans.[15] In another study that compared rigid immigration policies and mental health in the Latinx community, Latinx people residing in states with stringent immigration policies experienced a greater number of poorer mental health days.[16] In summary, mental health disparities are longstanding, widely prevalent, and deeply problematic.

Disparities in Substance Use Disorders

Addiction to drugs or alcohol comprises a mental illness known as SUD. SUD is defined as a problematic pattern of substance use that causes significant impairment or distress.[17] SUD are shaped by genetic, environmental, and developmental factors, leading to an array of mental, physical, and behavioral symptoms.[18] A subset of SUD is opioid use disorder (OUD). The term opioid is used to describe a class of drugs that includes prescription pain relievers, synthetic opioids, and heroin.[19] OUD carries a great possibility of developing a physical dependence in a short timeframe, sometimes as little as 4 weeks—and abruptly stopping opioid use can lead to severe withdrawal symptoms.[20] Because mental health and SUD are closely tied together, similar disparities exist among minority populations. African Americans and Latinx populations are less likely to complete treatment for SUD, because psychosocial stressors and the severity of drug use are cited as influences on the completion of treatment.[21] Compared with whites, Latinx populations have a 92% likelihood of completing treatment for substance abuse and African Americans have a 69% likelihood.[8] African Americans are also less likely to complete treatment across several substances, including alcohol, cocaine, marijuana, heroin, and methamphetamine compared with whites.[8]

Not only do minority groups have lower rates of treatment completion, but they are also less likely to receive treatment at all. OUD is now considered a public health emergency as more than 130 Americans die daily as a result of this crisis.[22] One of the most beneficial evidence-based treatments for OUD involves medications for addiction treatment (MAT). MAT is the use of medications in combination with counseling and behavioral therapies; it is proven to be effective in the treatment of opioid use and in helping to sustain recovery.[23] Buprenorphine, methadone, and naltrexone are the 3 drugs that have been approved by the US Food and Drug Administration to fight opioid dependence.[23] Typically, these treatments have been most effective when combined with counseling and psychosocial support.[23] From 2004 to 2015, buprenorphine was more likely to be provided to patients that were white, had private insurance, and/or could self-pay.[4] Research shows that, between 2012 and 2015, there were a total of 13.4 million patient visits that resulted in a buprenorphine prescription; white patients accounted for 95% of those visits and minority patients accounted for only about 3%.[24] Further, for every 35 white patients who received a buprenorphine prescription, 1 minority patient did, with an overall 77% lower odds of having an office visit that included a buprenorphine prescription.[24] Race and class are inextricably linked, making race, ethnicity, and income defining aspects of access. Between 2012 and 2015, approximately 40% of outpatient visits involving buprenorphine prescriptions were paid for by the patient outside of insurance, with private insurance covering only 34% of these costs, and only 19% were paid for by either Medicare or Medicaid.[24] Although 69% of counties in the United States have at least 1 SUD facility, about 40% do not have at least 1 outpatient SUD facility that accepts Medicaid.[25] Counties in the South and Midwest, as well as those with higher proportions of African American and/or Latinx residents, were less likely to have SUD outpatient facilities that accept Medicaid.[25]

Amid the OUD epidemic, several barriers hinder treatment for co-occurring disorders, including personal beliefs (ie, perceived stigma, cultural attitudes) and structural barriers (ie, insurance coverage, service availability and location, disorder identification, and lack of provider training to identify the disorders).[26] There is a lack of specialized services for treatment for substance abuse and mental health, particularly in rural areas.[26] Further, research suggests that negative stereotypes may contribute to the underdiagnoses and misdiagnoses of racial, ethnic, gender, and sexual minorities.[26] As the number of Americans with SUD grows, there is a pressing need to increase access to treatment for black, Latinx, and low-income populations to ensure all who could benefit from this treatment are provided appropriate access.

THE COST OF MENTAL HEALTH AND SUBSTANCE USE DISORDERS

Mental health care costs the United States about $300 billion annually, including $100 billion in health care expenditures.[27,28] Mental disorders are considered some of the highest cost medical conditions, with spending having increased by 5.6% between 1996 and 2013.[28] When substance use is taken into account, mental health and SUD services combined account for 7% of overall health care spending in 2014.[29] Medicare and Medicaid covered more than one-half of all spending on mental health care and SUD services, totaling $110 billion and $22 billion, respectively.[29] Early recognition and treatment of mental illness can lead to a decreased number of medical visits, ultimately decreasing costs. Further, mental illness increases the likelihood of morbidity for several chronic diseases, including cardiovascular diseases, obesity, diabetes, and cancer.[27] This finding suggests that providing accessible and high-quality treatments has the potential to improve outcomes for chronic diseases, further decreasing health care expenditures.[27] Eliminating mental health disparities by providing additional care can lead to the United States saving up to $38 million in emergency room expenditures and $833 million in inpatient expenditures for black and Latinx populations.[30] These significant cost decreases indicate an urgency to promote mental health and SUD equity. The World Health Organization states that investing in mental health is key to the advancement of and well-being of populations and improves economic efficiency.[31] The World Health Organization lists 4 ways to begin this investment:

1. Increase awareness and education about mental health and illness.
2. Provide better quality health and social care services for underserved populations with unmet needs.
3. Provide better social and financial protection for persons with mental disorders, particularly those in socially disadvantaged groups.

4. Provide better legislative protection and social support for persons, families, and communities adversely affected by mental disorders.[31]

These investment areas highlight the need for interventions that address equity not only at the individual and community level, but the structural level as well.

MENTAL HEALTH PARITY AND SUBSTANCE USE DISORDER EQUITY

The Mental Health Parity and Addiction Equity Act, which was enacted in 2008, requires that, when mental health or SUD benefits are covered, they are covered equally with physical health services.[32] SUD treatment is an essential health benefit for individual and small group coverage under the Affordable Care Act.[33] Although the passing of this landmark law helped to ameliorate the bifurcation of mental health and physical health, mental health and SUD parity compliance remains a work in progress across public and commercial payers, despite having been the law for more than a decade.

Meaningful oversight and enforcement of mental health and SUD parity are critical to reversing the current opioid epidemic, yet legislation alone is not the solution. In addition to enforcement, the removal of barriers such as prior authorization for MAT services, ensuring that MAT is affordable, and that health insurance companies have an adequate network of addiction medicine and mental health physicians are also crucial to addressing disparities in treatment. The business case has to be made at the intersection of regulators, payers, and providers who need appropriate incentives for investment. Both payers and health systems have become adept at adhering to the letter of the law, balancing regulatory requirements with financial restraints in deciding how to respond to shifts in regulations. Consequently, an ecosystem approach that accounts for the multiple and varied incentives of key stakeholders to address mental health and SUD is required and tangible; meaningful data must be acquired and disseminated.

MAKING THE BUSINESS CASE: REAL-WORLD EVIDENCE TRIALS

Traditional clinical trials, although of great value, are costly and time consuming, often spanning multiple years in development and navigating the complex approval process. Moreover, clinical trials are often conducted with specific populations, controlled in certain environments that do not reflect clinical or community realities.[34] Historically, clinical trials have struggled to have diverse participants and have, at times, increased disparities by focusing their studies on discrete populations.[34] Real-world evidence trials have the potential to compensate for the limitations of traditional clinical trials, improving the ability to generalize findings to be more inclusive of diverse populations.[34] This allows researchers to answer questions that better pertain to these populations, gaining a deeper understanding of how clinical settings, providers, and health systems affect treatments and outcomes. Real-world evidence trials involve information gathered beyond typical clinical research settings (ie, electronic health records, claims and billing data, disease registries, data from health informatics, personal devices, and health applications).[34] Thus, although efficacy trials aim to understand whether an intervention leads to a certain result under ideal conditions, effectiveness trials seek to assess the degree of effect under real-world clinical settings that are often impacted by factors such as patient preference, organization culture, administrative decisions, and organizational structure of the entities involved.[35] Real-world evidence trials, which embrace a health ecosystem approach and account for multiple entities and diverse incentives, could uncover financial, operational, and strategic factors required to enhance the business case for meaningful investment in mental health and SUD.

Enhancing the business case using real-world evidence trials in mental health and SUD would best be served by incorporating a health ecosystem approach and collaborating with appropriate payers, health systems, and related parties in the recovery ecosystem, including those involved in outpatient care, inpatient care, housing, and social support services. Collecting and analyzing patient outcomes and financial outcomes could offer a data-driven and strategic opportunity to compel investment in mental health and SUD. For example, regarding OUD, strategic questions to answer would include the following: Does reducing the barriers to access, such as prior authorization of MAT, lead to fewer overdose deaths? Does reducing barriers save payers and health systems money when compared with the cost of overdose in the emergency room and other high-cost settings? Does the costlier injectable extended-release version of buprenorphine lead to fewer hospitalizations and emergency room admissions than the less expensive oral buprenorphine, and ultimately save more despite the higher upfront costs of injectable medications? Providing the answers to such trenchant questions in a real-world setting with a lens toward operational, financial, and patient outcomes could form a cogent argument for investing in OUD, and mental health and SUD more broadly, in minority communities.

MAKING THE BUSINESS CASE: MEDICAID AND REAL-WORLD EVIDENCE

Medicaid is both a federal and state program that provides health insurance for low-income individuals, and is one of the largest purchasers of health care services in the United States, providing coverage for more than 70 million people at an annual cost of more than $460 billion.[36] Medicaid is also the largest payer for mental health services in the United States and generally the first or second largest item in every state budget.[37] Given that Medicaid is a program for the poor and largely serves Latinx and black populations, Medicaid could act as the epicenter for rapidly addressing disparities in mental health and SUD access and treatment. Medicaid's size, scope, and centrality in the health insurance market make it a viable opportunity. Historically, for Medicaid, cost containment has meant imposing arbitrary across-the-board rate cuts or cutting eligibility, but the time is ripe for state Medicaid agencies to leverage real-world evidence trials.

Unlike Medicare, which is managed across the country under central administration, each state Medicaid office has latitude regarding how they administer the program. This latitude presents both a challenge and an opportunity. Coverage policy, in its broadest sense, is intended to promote value in medical care by using reimbursement to favor the use of effective care and avoid payment for ineffective care.[38]

Ways in which Medicaid can address disparities become apparent when exploring mental health and OUD treatment. For example, all state Medicaid offices are required to pay for mental health inpatient stays, but optional benefit categories include effective evidence-based nonclinical services such as peer support and community residential services and vary greatly by state.[37] On a more granular level, although all state Medicaid offices offer coverage for buprenorphine, which is used in MAT, 40 states require prior authorization for its use.[39] In a similar vein, Medicaid coverage for extended-release injectable buprenorphine is covered by 33 state Medicaid offices but only 7 do not require prior authorization.[40] Prior authorization is an effective tactic to prevent overuse and manage costs, but it has also been proven to be a barrier to care particularly for minority communities.[4] Real-world evidence trials could be a powerful tool to study financial and patient data, connecting the decrease of prior authorization requirements to the decrease in overdose deaths and expensive emergency room visits associated with overdose. Similarly, real-world evidence trials could determine the impact of oral buprenorphine and the extended-release injectable buprenorphine and analyze cost differentials and overdose rates based on geography, health system characteristics, and race and ethnicity. Data-driven decision making based on patient and financial data in real-world settings could positively impact the opioid crisis, decrease costs, and meaningfully address disparities in mental health and SUD.

PRIVATE SECTOR INVESTMENT

There are instances of local communities across the country taking this leap; communities in Kansas and Colorado have now passed local taxes to build their capacity to address mental health and SUD.[41,42] In private industry, the Google affiliate, Verily, in Dayton, Ohio—considered the epicenter of the OUD crisis—established a nonprofit organization called OneFifteen to highlight and address the 115 people who die daily from OUD.[43] Additionally, private foundations in different states, including the Colorado Health Foundation, are now offering zero interest loans to inspire investment in mental health as well as in mental health innovation and technologies.[44,45] Although community investment in mental health and OUD is promising, more remains to be done at the payor, provider, state, and federal levels to address the OUD epidemic and decrease disparities in access and treatment to mental health and SUD services more broadly.

SUMMARY

The cost of our nation's mental health and SUD burden continues to escalate and is further exacerbated by health disparities that impact minority and low-income populations. Acknowledging the business case for addressing our mental health and SUD crisis is of vital importance. Although there are no easy answers, it is incumbent upon health systems, policymakers, and payers to address the human and financial cost of this crisis. A health ecosystem approach that aligns disparate incentives and accounts for financial, operational, and strategic concerns of payers and health systems is needed to inspire investment in mental health and SUD in underserved communities across the country. Although the human cost of the mental health and SUD epidemic is clear, navigating the "whose pockets" issue of cost decreases associated with these investments remains a challenge. Real-world evidence trials, which account for strategic and operational concerns along with the disparate financial incentives of multiple stakeholders, offer great promise to reduce disparities and combat this major challenge of our generation.

DISCLOSURE

The authors have nothing to disclose.

REFERENCES

1. National Alliance on Mental Illness. Mental health by the numbers. 2019. Available at: https://www.nami.org/learn-more/mental-health-by-the-numbers. Accessed December 23, 2019.
2. American Addiction Centers. Alcohol and drug abuse statistics. 2020. Available at: https://americanaddictioncenters.org/rehab-guide/addiction-statistics. Accessed December 28, 2019.

3. Wang PS, Lane M, Olfson M, et al. Twelve-month use of mental health services in the United States: results from the national comorbidity survey replication. Arch Gen Psychiatry 2005;62(6):629–40.

4. Lagisetty P, Ross R, Bohnert A. Buprenorphine treatment divide by race/ethnicity and payment. JAMA Psychiatry 2019;76(9):979–81.

5. Cook BL, Zuvekas SH, Carson N, et al. Assessing racial/ethnic disparities in treatment across episodes of mental health care. Health Serv Res 2014;49(1):206–29.

6. Alegria M, Page JB, Hansen H, et al. Improving drug treatment services for Hispanics: research gaps and scientific opportunities. Drug and Alcohol Depend 2006;84S:S76–84.

7. Guerrero EG, Marsh JC, Khachikian T, et al. Disparities in Latino substance use, service use, and treatment: implications for culturally and evidence-based interventions under health care reform. Drug and Alcohol Depend 2013;133:805–13.

8. Mennis J, Stahler GJ. Racial and ethnic disparities in outpatient substance use disorder treatment episode completion for different substances. J Subst Abuse Treat 2016;63:25–33.

9. Substance Abuse and Mental Health Services Administration. Racial/ethnic differences in mental health service use among adults. Rockville (MD): Substance Abuse and Mental Health Services Administration; 2015.

10. Sentell T, Shumway M, Snowden L. Access to mental health treatment by English language proficiency and race/ethnicity. J Gen Intern Med 2007;22:289–93.

11. Safran MA, Mays RA Jr, Huang LN, et al. Mental health disparities. Am J Public Health 2009;99(11):1962–6.

12. Institute of Medicine. Unequal treatment: confronting racial and ethnic disparities in health care. Washington, DC: The National Academies Press; 2003.

13. Compton MT, Shim RS. The social determinants of mental health focus. J Lifelong Learn Psychiatry 2015;13(4):419–25.

14. Mojtabai R, Olfson M, Sampson NA, et al. Barriers to mental health treatment: results from the national comorbidity survey replication (NCS-R). Psychol Med 2011;41(8):1751–61.

15. Hatzenbuehler ML, McLaughlin KA, Keyes KM, et al. The impact of institutional discrimination on psychiatric disorders in lesbian, gay, and bisexual populations: a prospective study. Am J Public Health 2010;100(3):452–9.

16. Hatzenbuehler ML, Prins S, Flake M, et al. Immigration policies and mental health morbidity among Latinos: a state-level analysis. Soc Sci Med 2017;174:169–78.

17. Center for Disease Control and Prevention. CDC guideline for prescribing opioids for chronic pain — United States. Atlanta, GA: CDC; 2016. p. 2016.

18. Volkow ND, Koob GF, McLellan AT. Neurobiologic advances from the brain disease model of addiction. N Engl J Med 2016;374(4):363–71.

19. National Institute on Drug Abuse. Opioids. Available at: https://www.drugabuse.gov/drugs-abuse/opioids. Accessed December 26, 2019.

20. American Psychiatric Association. Opioid use disorder. 2018. Available at: https://www.psychiatry.org/patients-families/addiction/opioid-use-disorder/opioid-use-disorder. Accessed December 20, 2019.

21. Guerrero EG, Marsh JC, Duan L, et al. Disparities in completion of substance abuse treatment between and within racial and ethnic groups. Health Serv Res 2013;48(4):1450–67.

22. National Institute on Drug Abuse. Opioid overdose crisis. 2019. Available at: https://www.drugabuse.gov/drugs-abuse/opioids/opioid-overdose-crisis. Accessed January 2, 2020.

23. US Food & Drug Administration. Information about Medication-Assisted Treatment (MAT). Information about Medication-Assisted Treatment (MAT). 2019. Available at: https://www.fda.gov/drugs/information-drug-class/information-about-medication-assisted-treatment-mat. Accessed January, 2020.
24. Robeznieks A. Black patients less likely to get treatment for opioid-use disorder. Chicago, IL: American Medical Association; 2019.
25. Cummings JR, Wen H, Ko M, et al. Race/ethnicity and geographic access to Medicaid substance use disorder treatment facilities in the United States. JAMA Psychiatry 2014;71(2):190–6.
26. Priester MA, Browne T, Iachini A, et al. Treatment access barriers and disparities among individuals with co-occurring mental health and substance use disorders: an integrative literature review. J Subst Abuse Treat 2015;61:47–59.
27. Reeves WC, Strine TW, Pratt LA, et al. Mental illness surveillance among adults in the United States. Atlanta (GA): Office of Surveillance, Epidemiology, and Laboratory Services, Centers for Disease Control and Prevention, U.S. Department of Health and Human Services; 2011.
28. Roehrig C. Mental disorders top the list of the most costly conditions in The United States: $201 Billion. Health Aff 2016;35(6):1130–5.
29. National Conference of State Legislatures. The costs and consequences of disparities in behavioral health care. 2018. Available at: http://www.ncsl.org/Portals/1/HTML_LargeReports/DisparitiesBehHealth_Final.htm. Accessed December 27, 2019.
30. Cook BL, Liu Z, Lessios AS, et al. The costs and benefits of reducing racial-ethnic disparities in mental health care. Psychiatr Serv 2015;66(4):389–96.
31. Chisholm D. Investing in mental health: evidence for action. Switzerland: World Health Organization; 2013.
32. Creedon TB, Cook BL. Access to mental health care increased but not for substance use, while disparities remain. Health Aff 2016;35(6):1017–21.
33. The Center for Consumer Information & Insurance Oversight. Information on Essential Health Benefits (EHB) benchmark plans. Available at: https://www.cms.gov/CCIIO/Resources/Data-Resources/ehb. Accessed January 3, 2020.
34. Sherman R, Anderson S, Pan GD, et al. Real-world evidence — what is it and what can it tell us? N Engl J Med 2016;375(23):2293–7.
35. Gartlehner G, Hansen RA, Nissman D, et al. Criteria for distinguishing effectiveness from efficacy trials in systematic reviews. Rockville (MD): Agency for Healthcare Research and Quality (US); 2006.
36. Clemans-Cope L, Holahan J, Garfield R. Medicaid spending growth compared to other payers: a look at the evidence. San Francisco, CA: Kaiser Commission on Medicaid and the Uninsured; 2016.
37. Musumeci M, Chidambaram P, Orgera K. State options for Medicaid coverage of inpatient behavioral health services. San Francisco, CA: Kaiser Family Foundation; 2019.
38. Garber AM. Evidence-based coverage policy. Health Aff (Millwood) 2001;20(5):62–82.
39. Weber E, Gupta A. State Medicaid programs should follow the "Medicare model": remove prior authorization requirements for buprenorphine and other medications to treat opioid use disorders. Washington, DC: Legal Action Center; 2019.
40. Substance Abuse and Mental Health Services Administration. Medicaid coverage of medication-assisted treatment for alcohol and opioid use disorders and of medication for the reversal of opioid overdose. Rockville (MD): Substance Abuse and Mental Health Services Administration; 2018.

41. Jones E. Voters overwhelmingly approve sales tax to fund behavioral health campus, services. 2018. Available at: https://www2.ljworld.com/news/county-government/2018/nov/06/voters-overwhelmingly-approve-sales-tax-to-fund-behavioral-health-campus-services/. Accessed January, 2020.

42. Benzel L. Local voters could hold key in Colorado's mental health crisis. The Gazette. Mental Health: A Crisis in Colorado Web site. 2019. Available at: https://gazette.com/premium/local-voters-could-hold-key-in-colorado-s-mental-health/article_98d74afa-16d9-11ea-b3b8-0f4a2928a97e.html. Accessed January, 2020.

43. Lester N. OneFifteen opens the first of its state-of-the-art facilities for the treatment of opioid use disorder in Dayton, Ohio. 2019. Available at: https://onefifteen.org/press/. Accessed January 3, 2020.

44. The Colorado Health Foundation. Funding opportunity: strengthening primary care. Available at: https://www.coloradohealth.org/funding-opportunities/funding-opportunity-strengthening-primary-care. Accessed March 31, 2020.

45. The Colorado Health Foundation. Colorado Health Foundation Announces groundbreaking investment with Denver-based, for-profit behavioral health app developer. Available at: https://coloradohealth.org/news/colorado-health-foundation-announces-groundbreaking-investment-denver-based-profit-behavioral. Accessed March 31, 2020.

Shifting the Policy Paradigm to Achieve Equity

Steven M. Starks, MD[a],*, Sidney H. Hankerson, MD, MBA[b],
Pamela Y. Collins, MD, MPH[c,d]

KEYWORDS

- Health policy • Health equity • Racial disparities • Health disparities
- Minority mental health • Advocacy • Mental health policy

KEY POINTS

- The foundations of the mental health system were rooted in inequality.
- Achieving mental health equity is a modern approach that confronts longstanding discriminatory policies.
- Major advances in mental health equity have occurred through policies that support research, improve access, and address barriers for racial and ethnic minorities.
- The path to achieve equity could occur by using community-informed policymaking.

INTRODUCTION

The preceding articles in this issue highlight the inequities that persist in mental health access, service delivery, and financing for groups designated as racial and ethnic minorities. In this article, we review the historical context of mental health policies, their impact on individuals and communities, and the barriers they present to ensuring comprehensive and equitable care for all. We describe social changes and activism that challenged the status quo to broaden the role of government in providing treatment and services for those with mental illness. Although we recognize the interplay of institutional, local, state, and national mental health policies in the promotion of equity and reform, here we direct our attention to federal policies that are the basis for the funding, infrastructure, and programming of the US mental health system. In addition, we examine the guiding principles that propel policymaking to target mental health

[a] Department of Clinical Sciences, University of Houston College of Medicine, Health 2 Building, 4849 Calhoun Road, Room 6014, Houston, TX 77201-6064, USA; [b] Columbia University, Vagelos College of Physicians and Surgeons, New York State Psychiatric Institute, 1051 Riverside Drive, New York, NY 10032, USA; [c] Department of Psychiatry and Behavioral Sciences, University of Washington Schools of Medicine and Public Health, 1959 Northeast Pacific Street, Box 356560, Seattle, WA 98195-6560, USA; [d] Department of Global Health, University of Washington Schools of Medicine and Public Health, 1959 Northeast Pacific Street, Box 356560, Seattle, WA 98195-6560, USA
* Corresponding author.
E-mail address: sstarks@central.uh.edu

Psychiatr Clin N Am 43 (2020) 439–450
https://doi.org/10.1016/j.psc.2020.05.004
0193-953X/20/© 2020 Elsevier Inc. All rights reserved.

equity. We consider contributing factors and current challenges to steady improvements in access and service delivery. Finally, we offer a structured model for policy development that is aligned with community-partnered participatory research that builds on community insights and strengths. We posit that a community-informed policy approach targets the key values of racial and ethnic minority groups and best sustains equity in mental health service utilization.

A HISTORICAL PERSPECTIVE ON MENTAL HEALTH POLICY AND RACE-BASED INEQUITY

Reflecting on policies related to the treatment of those with mental illnesses and the origins of American medical practice provides a useful lens to examine our current state of health disparities. Race has been uniquely intertwined with the mental health system since its inception. In fact, the enslavement of African American individuals was purported to be a protective factor for their mental health. Erroneous reporting in the mid-nineteenth century estimated that the prevalence of mental illnesses among African American individuals residing in free states was more than 10 times that of those residing in states with enslavement.[1] This propaganda not only argued against abolitionist and emancipation movements at that time, but also impacted local and state government responses and philanthropic support needed to apply resources in the care of those experiencing mental illness. These trends continued after the Civil War, Emancipation, and Reconstruction periods, as segregation pervaded the mental health services landscape. Local municipalities and state governments provided custodial care and treatment of African American individuals in separate institutions or wards. In a similar manner to "separate but equal" facilities and resources in education and housing systems, institutional and custodial care for African American individuals was largely inaccessible, scant, or of poorer quality.[2,3]

For Native American individuals, a segregated health care system also existed. Despite a federal trust relationship since our nation's establishment (ie, one built on formal agreements, treaties, and law), tribal lands received minimal resources and funding from the Bureau of Indian Affairs to support their health needs.[4] In the 1920s, there was only one hospital in existence for the treatment of Native American individuals with mental illness.[5] A 1928 report to the US Secretary of the Interior by the Institute on Government Research, known as the Meriam Report, assessed the administration of resources to tribes. The document detailed the poor health and living conditions of Native American individuals.[5] Its findings concluded that the infrastructure and workforce were far too inadequate to meet the expected needs of tribal territories, a circumstance that persists today.[6]

The twentieth century ushered in a national response to mental health care and a confluence of social policies that advanced ideals of equality (**Table 1**). The National Mental Health Act was signed into law in 1946 and served as an answer to strained public health services and resources in the wake of World War II. As the mental health workforce addressed the needs of military service members and veterans, significant gaps remained in state hospitals, correctional institutions, immigration services, and drug addiction services.[7] Although this Act spurred federal programs aimed at research, prevention, and workforce development, it failed to address the needs of African American veterans and communities.[8,9] Latinx veterans additionally faced racial discrimination post-War.[10] The legislation's provisions would ultimately direct funding to the development of the National Institute of Mental Health (NIMH).

During the 1940s and 1950s, proponents of the rehabilitation and civil liberties movements decried the abusive and unsanitary conditions of state mental hospitals.

Table 1
Shifts in national policy that impacted equity in mental health

Year	Driver of Policy Shift	Behavioral Response to Policy Shift
1946	National Mental Health Act	Authorized services, research, training for mental health; established National Institute for Mental Health (NIMH)
1963	Mental Retardation Facilities and Community Mental Health Centers Construction Act	Established community mental health programs; contributed to deinstitutionalization; contributed to transinstitutionalization to nursing homes and criminal justice involvement
1964	Civil Rights Act, Title VI (preceded by *Simkins v. Cone*)	Prohibited discrimination in federally funded programs
1965	Medicare/Medicaid	Desegregated hospitals and health care systems
1970	Nixon Administration's Establishment of the NIMH Center for Minority Group Mental Health Programs	Stimulated research and training support to combat racism
1980	Mental Health Systems Act	Designated an NIMH associate director of minority concerns for services, research, training and workforce programming
1985	U. S. Dept. of Health and Human Services (HHS) Report of the Secretary's Task Force on Black and Minority Health (Heckler Report)	Led to creation of the HHS Office of Minority Health
1986	State Comprehensive Mental Health Services Plan Act	Impacted provision of case management services and community-based systems of care
2001	*Mental Health: Culture, Race and Ethnicity* (Surgeon General's Report)	Offered a roadmap to achieve mental health equity
2008	Mental Health Parity & Addiction Equity Act	Application of standards for mental health and addiction insurance benefits that were equitable to other medical benefits
2010	Patient Protection and Affordable Care Act	Expanded access to health coverage through Medicaid expansion and insurance definitions and subsidies; expanded minority health impacts within key federal agencies

In response to public outcry, advancements in biological treatments, and community-based rehabilitation movements, the Community Mental Health Centers Act (1963) shepherded national reforms to develop community-based mental health services. States were granted federal funds to serve local catchment areas and provided inpatient, outpatient, and education services and treatment.[11] Whether by design or unintentional, catchment areas segregated communities. An individual from a racial-minority community received care at a designated facility defined solely by catchment, which contributed to stereotyping and disparities in services and treatment.[12] Further advances in the Civil Rights Movement propelled mental health for racial and ethnic minorities. The federal appeals court decisions that instituted nondiscrimination in hospitals receiving federal funding were fully mandated through Title VI of the Civil Rights Act of 1964.[13] Through amendments of the Social Security Act, the Medicare and Medicaid programs (1965) led to the desegregation of hospitals and health care systems.

TWENTIETH CENTURY POLICIES TO ADDRESS MINORITY MENTAL HEALTH

The violent and tumultuous social fabric of the late 1960s placed racism at the forefront of societal plagues requiring immediate attention. The National Advisory Commission on Civil Disorders (ie, the Kerner Commission[14]) described racism as the primary cause of violence in the country and the Joint Commission on Mental Health of Children, Inc.[15] defined racism as the primary public health problem in America. African American psychiatrists and mental health professions engaged in federal advocacy to support improved service delivery to minority communities. In response, NIMH established the Center for Minority Group Mental Health Programs[16] (1970–1985) to improve research efforts and workforce development.

The first major charge to legislate racial equity in mental health came through the Mental Health Systems Act of 1980 (Public Law 96–398), which designated an Associate Director of Minority Concerns at NIMH. The associate director would oversee services and programs for minority groups and direct programs for researching and training, and workforce initiatives. Although other key provisions of this Act were repealed in the subsequent change in administration, this position endured.[17] The 1985 Department of Health and Human Services (HHS) report on Black and Minority Health, known as the Heckler Report,[18] critically detailed the differences in multiple health outcomes for minority groups and spurred a federal response and commitment to examining racial disparities. The Heckler Report inspired the creation of the HHS Office of Minority Health. In 1992, Public Law 102 to 321 would establish the NIMH Associate Director for Special Populations, a role charged with coordinating research policies and programs to ensure emphasis on the needs of women and minority populations.

President Ronald Reagan's policy of New Federalism aimed to reduce the size and influence of the federal government.[19] In effect, it curtailed social programs and entitlements that provided economic, employment, and housing support to communities in need. This fiscal conservatism affected minority groups, those in poverty, and people with mental illnesses the most.[20] The 1980s also heralded a shift in the health finance system with the introduction of managed care plans, expansions in mental health benefits, and new policies directing payments for mental health services. One example is the State Comprehensive Mental Health Services Plan Act that focused on supporting community-based systems of care and those psychosocial services integral to mental health treatment such as case management.[21] The Act stressed the need for care for all people with severe mental illnesses and for new research and service delivery plans for homeless people with chronic mental illnesses.

Overall, the progression of national reforms during the twentieth century resulted in the advancement of federal oversight, the implementation of national mental health programming, and the transition of care and services from state mental hospitals to federally sponsored programs like nursing homes and prisons, or community-based systems of care.[21] The interconnectedness of health and social services placed greater emphasis on solutions to enhance policies for both. As diagnoses and treatments were refined and definitions of mental illness broadened beyond severe, chronic illnesses, the importance of mental health for our society became more notable, and policies to ensure equity and parity of mental health benefits (equal to those for physical health) led the next wave of reforms. Although growing evidence showed racial and ethnic disparities in mental health care and outcomes, and a foundation had been established with NIMH programming aimed at racial and ethnic groups, few policies proposed significant actions to improve access and promote equity for minority populations.

A shift from institutional to community services had significant consequences for minority communities. The concept of *deinstitutionalization*, defined as the reintegration of individuals from state mental hospitals into their communities to receive community-based treatments, failed for many. For certain segments of society, community-based treatments for severe mental illness were often unavailable and inaccessible. As a result, *transinstitutionalization*, or the transfer of individuals from state mental hospitals to other institutions, occurred instead. These settings were typically ill-equipped to provide adequate, high-quality mental health services. Justice involvement through incarceration particularly plagued African American individuals, because the combination of race, socioeconomic status, and the distressing behaviors associated with severe mental illness often led to legal consequences.[22–24]

A TWENTY-FIRST CENTURY APPROACH TO PROMOTING EQUITY IN MENTAL HEALTH POLICY

In August 2001, the 16th US Surgeon General, Dr David Satcher, released the seminal report on disparities in mental health. Although not a policy document, *Mental Health: Culture, Race and Ethnicity*[25] outlined the strategy for achieving equity in the American health care system. This supplement to a broader document, *Mental Health: a Report of the Surgeon General*,[26] outlined the mental health needs of specific racial and ethnic group members, described the differences in access to services for these groups, and detailed the disparate outcomes in care for African American, American Indian, Asian American, Pacific Islander, and Hispanic American individuals. It delineated a public health approach to ensuring equity for all through advancing research, improving access to high-quality care, and promoting mental health through workforce development and consumer/community engagement (**Box 1**). In the following year, the Institute of Medicine's consensus report, *Unequal Treatment*,[27] on racial and ethnic disparities in health care echoed this approach. Incremental shifts in policy occurred as a result, including quality improvement through national standards for culturally and linguistically appropriate services.[28]

In the context of growing rates of unmet mental health service needs, advances in achieving parity for mental health care occurred nearly a decade later, with the passage of the Mental Health Parity and Addiction Equity Act of 2008 (MHPAEA), which was implemented in January 2010. The MHPAEA had mixed effects on equity. People with common mental disorders like depression were more likely to be treated in primary care; however, non-Hispanic African American individuals were less likely to receive care.[29]

The passage of the Affordable Care Act (ACA) in March 2010 conferred the largest advances in access to benefits and services for racial/ethnic minorities. The major provisions[30] expanded insurance access through increases in income limits for Medicaid eligibility, subsidies for insurance premiums for low earners, coverage of young adults up to age 26 on their parents' insurance plans, and inclusion of mental health benefits under its mandated essential health benefits coverage. Some lesser-known provisions made key changes within federal government departments and agencies (**Box 2**): the promotion of the Office of Minority Health within HHS, the elevation of the National Center on Minority Health and Health Disparities to a National Institutes of Health

---

Box 1
Sixteenth surgeon general's suggested approach to address inequity in mental health

Continue to Expand the Science Base
- Epidemiology
- Evidence-based treatment
- Psychopharmacology
- Ethnic- or culture-specific interventions
- Diagnosis and assessment
- Prevention and promotion
- Study the roles of culture, race, and ethnicity in mental health

Improve Access to Treatment
- Improve geographic access
- Integrate mental health and primary care
- Ensure language access
- Coordinate and integrate mental health services for high-need populations

Reduce Barriers to Treatment
- Ensure parity and expand public health insurance
- Extend health insurance for the uninsured
- Examine the costs and benefits of culturally appropriate services
- Reduce barriers to managed care
- Overcome shame, stigma, and discrimination
- Build trust in mental health services

Improve Quality of Care
- Ensure evidence-based treatment
- Develop and evaluate culturally responsive services
- Engage consumers, families, and communities in developing services

Support Capacity Development
- Train mental health professionals
- Encourage consumer and family leadership

Promote Mental Health
- Address social adversities
- Build on natural support
- Strengthen families

Data from Office of the Surgeon General, Center for Mental Health, National Institute of Mental Health, et al. Mental Health: Culture, Race, and Ethnicity—A Supplement to Mental Health: A Report of the Surgeon General. Rockville, MD: Department of Health and Human Services; 2001.

Institute, and the formation of minority health offices in targeted federal agencies that oversee research, epidemiology, health care finance, drug innovation and safety, workforce and resources, and mental health and substance use programs. With a primary aim of ensuring more Americans had comprehensive health care coverage, the ACA bridged significant gaps in health equity; however, novel models in policymaking are still needed to sustain improvements in quality and capacity.

FUTURE DIRECTIONS: A MODEL OF COMMUNITY-INFORMED POLICYMAKING

One promising avenue for creating demand for policy change is community-based participatory research (CBPR). CBPR blends rigorous science with social activism.[31] CBPR methods equitably involve community members, health care providers, organizational representatives, academicians, and policymakers in the research process.[32] Most CBPR makes use of the social-ecological model of health, which considers how

---

Box 2
Provisions of the Affordable Care Act that improved equity in mental health

Transfer of the Office of Minority Health to the Office of the Health and Human Services Secretary

Establishment of individual Offices of Minority Health within the following agencies:
- Agency for Healthcare Research and Quality
- Centers for Disease Control and Prevention
- Centers for Medicare and Medicaid Services
- Food and Drug Administration
- Health Resources and Services Administration
- Substance Abuse and Mental Health Services Administration

Redesignation of the National Center on Minority Health and Health Disparities to an institute within the National Institutes of Health; that is, the National Institute on Minority Health and Health Disparities

Data from U.S. Department of Health and Human Services, Office of the Secretary, Office of Minority Health for the Fiscal Years 2013 and 2014 Report to Congress on Minority Health Activities as Required by the Patient Protection and Affordable Care Act (P.L. 111-148). Available at: https://minorityhealth.hhs.gov/Assets/pdf/2015_0916_Report_to_Congress_on_Minority_Health_Activities_FINAL.pdf.

---

policy, community, interpersonal, and individual-level factors contribute to health inequities.[33–35] Given its attention to multiple determinants of health, CBPR aims to achieve policy and broad-scale changes focused on health equity.[32]

Community-partnered participatory research (CPPR), derived from CBPR, can promote health equity in mental health services utilization. The core values of CPPR are respect for diversity, 2-way power-sharing, knowledge, trust, and community empowerment.[36] CPPR analyzes progress through 3 sequential phases: vision (engagement of stakeholders and collaborative planning), valley (implementation of evidence-based practices), and victory (celebration and communicating results).[37] A Community Steering Council composed of community members, policymakers, and academicians provide leadership for community-partnered initiatives.[38] In a landmark federally funded study, Community Partners in Care, a participatory approach was compared with technical assistance for quality depression care. This study assessed the effectiveness of implementing evidence-based depression interventions in underresourced communities in South Los Angeles, populations that were predominantly African American or Latinx.[39,40] Results showed that Community Partners in Care improved depression screening uptake and outcomes in health care and social sectors, including churches, when compared with technical assistance.[41] Long-term follow-up of participants in the 2 groups showed increased depression remission among people who received the participatory approach.[42] These findings show that CPPR-informed methods can create sustainable effects and models of mental health service provision.[42,43]

A MODEL OF COMMUNITY-INFORMED POLICYMAKING: CASE EXAMPLE
The Black Church

Defined as the set of 7 predominantly African American denominations of Christian faith, the Black Church is one of the most durable and trusted institutions in African American communities.[44] The Black Church has provided de facto mental health services for centuries.[45] Their clergy are trusted "gatekeepers" for counseling services or referrals to mental health specialists.[46] Clergy also refer parishioners to mental health services and may influence the acceptability of their use.[47]

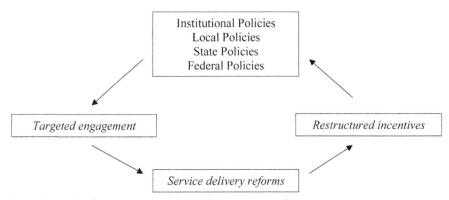

Fig. 1. Example of a community-informed policy approach.

The Black Church also has a storied history of engaging communities to shape policy. The most recognized illustration of its involvement in social justice was the Civil Rights Movement.[48] Integrating community-partnered approaches with the political force of the church could be a promising strategy to promote mental health equity. **Fig. 1** describes these approaches. Targeted engagement of congregations through education on mental health disparities and assessment of community mental health needs can inform advocacy for increased access to providers, more availability of service settings in local communities, or increased quality of care. Clergy trained in evidence-based psychosocial interventions or congregants equipped to provide peer support exemplify other modes of targeted engagement and service delivery. These changes in service delivery or delivery outcomes require restructured incentives that reward quality of care and deployment of diverse providers, including clergy. Value-based reimbursement options for mental health services provided by clergy or church-based paraprofessionals increase their likelihood of sustainability. Evidence of efficiency and cost-effectiveness mobilizes churches and community advocates to push for policies that support these new approaches to care. This community-informed approach serves the unique needs of its targeted population. In addition to applications in faith-based settings, this model could be adapted to confront the varying array of mental health policy needs of groups with diverse racial, ethnic, gender, or sexual identities (see **Fig. 1**).

DISCUSSION

Despite broad systemic improvements in health care, directing research, workforce, and services to enhance the mental health of racial and ethnic minorities remains a challenge. Social and economic policies that negatively affect minority communities contribute to disparities in health care utilization and outcomes. Despite growing public enthusiasm and approval of national policy proposals that would expand health care coverage for the uninsured, underinsured, or all Americans, there remains little momentum to promote reforms and enhancements of federal entitlement programs that confer economic, nutrition, or housing security (ie, key factors that influence health outcomes). Indeed, some markers of socioeconomic disadvantage (eg, lower neighborhood education) are associated with less initiation of mental health care.[49,50]

Major advances in mental health care financing have expanded benefit coverage and access to treatments and services, yet minority populations remain plagued by disparate and unequal care and outcomes. Among its many successes in attaining health equity, the ACA addressed a crucial disparity in health care for African American individuals, Latinx people, American Indian/Alaska Native peoples, and Native Hawaiian individuals: that of insurance coverage. Before full implementation of the ACA, the uninsured rates for adults were 19%, 30%, 30%, and 18%, respectively (compared with 12% for white individuals) in 2013. Four years later, in 2017, uninsured rates decreased significantly (11%, 19%, 22%, and 11% respectively, compared with 7% for white individuals). Greater impacts in ACA insurance coverage for minority groups are seen in states that expanded Medicaid eligibility in comparison with nonexpansion states.[51,52] Unfortunately, access to insurance coverage may belie assurances of access to high-quality care or service utilization. Kim and colleagues[53] revealed significantly lower use of mental health services by African American seniors in the South compared with white seniors, yet showed no racial differences in other geographic regions. Furthermore, disparities in mental health care among African American individuals and Latinx people are greatest at the initiation of care (compared with middle and end-phases of care).[51,52] Tauler and colleagues[49] note that advocacy to influence health policies and social policies that reduce disadvantage should be pursued simultaneously with efforts to expand the delivery of clinical interventions. In effect, health equity strategies require a multipronged approach.

One important transformative task in achieving equity involves the use of health care analytics to examine aggregated data to uncover utilization rates and differences by race/ethnicity. These data might allow for culturally targeted strategies to promote mental health equity. Another opportunity lies in repairing historical mistrust tied to past discrimination. How could policies incentivize health care systems to engage minority populations, particularly for care initiation, where disparities are most apparent? The government could play a role through financial reforms in federal programs. Training and workforce development could be increased at the state and federal levels and mandate that all mental health professionals receive training to address health equity locally (if applicable based on geography and specific metrics). Specifically, this may require training to implement evidence-based interventions that show the most promise in supporting mental health service initiation among ethnic minority communities, like integrated models of care. Because community health centers play a significant role in the provision of services for racial and ethnic minorities, funding full development of integrated behavioral health models in these primary care settings should benefit their consumers. Regional and geographic disparities could be addressed through novel federal block grants to target underserved groups. Federally, provisions of the ACA have been under attack since its implementation. Protecting health insurance and subsidies for those who benefit from the law and expanding insurance for uninsured and underinsured is vital. Finally, optimization of policy interventions by local, state, and federal actors must be accompanied by collaborative inquiry that engages communities, clinicians, and researchers in research on the complex interventions to improve mental health equity.

DISCLOSURE

The authors have nothing to disclose.

REFERENCES

1. Jarvis E. ART V.–Insanity among the Coloured Population of the Free States. Am J Med Sci 1844;7(13):71.

2. Pearson RL. There Are Many Sick, Feeble, and Suffering Freedmen": The Freedmen's Bureau's Health-Care Activities during Reconstruction in North Carolina, 1865-1868. N C Hist Rev 2002;79(2):141–81.
3. Rabinowitz HN. From exclusion to segregation: health and welfare services for southern blacks, 1865-1890. Soc Serv Rev 1974;48(3):327–54.
4. Dyste A. It's hard out here for an American Indian: implications of the Patient Protection and Affordable Care Act for the American Indian population. Law Inequal 2014;32:95.
5. Meriam L, Work H. The problem of Indian administration: report of a survey made at the request of honorable Hubert Work, secretary of the interior, and submitted to him, February 21, 1928. Baltimore, MD: Johns Hopkins Press; 1928.
6. United States Commission on Civil R. Broken promises: evaluating the Native American health care system. Washington, DC: US Commission on Civil Rights; 2004.
7. Brand JL. The National Mental Health Act of 1946: a retrospect. Bull Hist Med 1965;39(3):231–45.
8. Spurlock J. Black psychiatrists and American psychiatry. Washington, DC: American Psychiatric Pub; 1999.
9. Kaplan M. Solomon Carter Fuller: where my caravan has rested. Lanham, MD: University Press of Amer; 2005.
10. Rosales S. Fighting the peace at home: Mexican American veterans and the 1944 GI Bill of Rights. Pac Hist Rev 2011;80(4):597–627.
11. Sharfstein SS. Whatever happened to community mental health? Psychiatr Serv 2000;51(5):616–20.
12. Turner CB, Kramer BM. Connections between racism and mental health. Mental health, racism, and sexism. Pittsburgh, PA: University of Pittsburgh Press; 1995:3-25. Available at: https://nam03.safelinks.protection.outlook.com/?url=https%3A%2F%2Fisbnsearch.org%2Fisbn%2F9780822955498&data=02%7C01%7Cj.surendrakumar%40elsevier.com%7C77d79faa032b4291272c08d8217bd936%7C9274ee3f94254109a27f9fb15c10675d%7C0%7C0%7C6372961 63581259247&sdata=SBRhK7ZLmJDopLk0VkDTfGv9UTiBdj0jRa%2BW%2BIQ PEk4%3D&reserved=0.
13. Reynolds PP. Professional and hospital discrimination and the US Court of Appeals Fourth Circuit 1956–1967. Am J Public Health 2004;94(5):710–20.
14. United States. National Advisory Commission on Civil D, Kerner O, Wicker T. Report of the national advisory commission on civil disorders: special introduction by Tom Wicker of the *New York Times*; [chairman, Otto Kerner]. Washington, DC: Bantam Books; 1968.
15. Joint Commission on Mental Health of Children. Crisis in child mental health: challenge for the 1970's; report. Washington, DC: Harper & Row; 1970.
16. Brown BS, Okura KP. A brief history of the Center for Minority Group Mental Health Programs at the National Institute of Mental Health. In: Willie CV, Reiker PP, Kramer BM, editors. Mental health, racism, and sexism. Pittsburgh (PA): University of Pittsburgh Press; 1995. p. 397–426.
17. Grob GN. Public policy and mental illnesses: Jimmy Carter's presidential commission on mental health. Milbank Q 2005;83(3):425–56.
18. Heckler M. Report of the Secretary's task force on Black & minority health. Washington, DC: US Department of Health and Human Services; 1985.
19. Reagan's 'new federalism'. Washington, DC: CQ Press; 1981. Available at: https://nam03.safelinks.protection.outlook.com/?url=http%3A%2F%2Flibrary. cqpress.com%2Fcqresearcher%2Fcqresrre1981040300&data=02%7C01%7Cj.

surendrakumar%40elsevier.com%7C77d79faa032b4291272c08d8217bd936%
7C9274ee3f94254109a27f9fb15c10675d%7C0%7C0%7C637296163581259247&
sdata=RriO%2BETWtkUdt5wsv4qXnzFiYd4hgvinIXMBKAqbWGo%3D&
reserved=0.

20. National Hispanic Heritage Week : the new federalism : impact on Hispanic health care. Rockville (MD): U.S. Dept. of Health, and Human Services, Public Health Services; 1982.

21. Grob GN. Mental health policy in America: myths and realities. Health Aff 1992; 11(3):7–22.

22. Prins SJ. Does transinstitutionalization explain the overrepresentation of people with serious mental illnesses in the criminal justice system? Community Ment Health J 2011;47(6):716–22.

23. White MC, Chafetz L, Collins-Bride G, et al. History of arrest, incarceration and victimization in community-based severely mentally ill. J Community Health 2006;31(2):123–35.

24. Anderson A, Von Esenwein S, Spaulding A, et al. Involvement in the criminal justice system among attendees of an urban mental health center. Health & Justice 2015;3(1):4.

25. Satcher D. Mental health: Culture, race, and ethnicity—a supplement to mental health: a report of the surgeon general. Washington, DC: US Department of Health and Human Services; 2001.

26. Satcher D. Mental health: a report of the surgeon general–executive summary. Prof Psychol Res Pract 2000;31(1):5.

27. Smedley BD, Stith AY, Nelson AR. Institute of Medicine, Committee on Understanding and Eliminating Racial and Ethnic Disparities in Health Care. Unequal treatment: confronting racial and ethnic disparities in healthcare. Washington, DC: National Academies Press; 2003.

28. Services USDoHaH. National standards for culturally and linguistically appropriate services in health care. Washington, DC: US Department of Health and Human Services. Office of Minority Health; 2001.

29. Goldberg DM, Lin H-C. Effects of the mental health parity and addictions equality act on depression treatment choice in primary care facilities. Int J Psychiatry Med 2017;52(1):34–47.

30. Protection P, Act AC. Patient protection and affordable care act. Public Law 2010; 111(48):759–62.

31. Israel BA, Eng E, Schulz AJ, et al, editors. Methods in community-based participatory research for health. San Francisco: Jossey-Bass; 2005.

32. Wallerstein N, Duran B, Oetzel JG, et al. Community-based participatory research for health: advancing social and health equity. San Francisco, CA: John Wiley & Sons; 2017.

33. Wells K, Miranda J, Bruce ML, et al. Bridging community intervention and mental health services research. Am J Psychiatry 2004;161(6):955–63.

34. Freudenberg N, Tsui E. Evidence, power, and policy change in community-based participatory research. Am J Public Health 2014;104(1):11–4.

35. Bronfenbrenner UJ. Ecological models of human development. In: Gauvain M, Cole M, editors. Readings on the development of children. New York, NY: Scientific American Books; vol. 2. 1994. p. 37–43.

36. Jones L, Wells K. Strategies for academic and clinician engagement in community-participatory partnered research. JAMA 2007;297(4):407–10.

37. Jones L, Wells K, Norris K, et al. The vision, valley, and victory of community engagement. Ethn Dis 2009;19(4 Suppl 6). S6-S3-7.

38. Jones L, Meade B, Forge N, et al. Begin your partnership: the process of engagement. Ethn Dis 2009;19(4 Suppl 6). S6-8-16.

39. Khodyakov D, Mendel P, Dixon E, et al. Community partners in care: leveraging community diversity to improve depression care for underserved populations. Int J Divers Organ Communities Nations 2009;9(2):167–81.

40. Chung B, Jones L, Dixon EL, et al, Community Partners in Care Steering Council. Using a community partnered participatory research approach to implement a randomized controlled trial: planning community partners in care. J Health Care Poor Underserved 2010;21(3):780–95.

41. Wells KB, Jones L, Chung B, et al. Community-partnered cluster-randomized comparative effectiveness trial of community engagement and planning or resources for services to address depression disparities. J Gen Intern Med 2013; 28(10):1268–78.

42. Arevian AC, Jones F, Tang L, et al. Depression remission from community coalitions versus individual program support for services: findings from Community Partners in Care, Los Angeles, California, 2010–2016. Am J Public Health 2019;109(S3):S205–13.

43. Hankerson SH, Wells K, Sullivan MA, et al. Partnering with African American churches to create a community coalition for mental health. Ethn Dis 2018; 28(Suppl 2):467–74.

44. Lincoln CE, Mamiya LH. The black church in the African American Experience. London: Duke University Press; 1990.

45. Blank MB, Mahmood M, Fox JC, et al. Alternative mental health services: the role of the black church in the South. Am J Public Health 2002;92(10):1668–72.

46. Hankerson SH, Watson KT, Lukachko A, et al. Ministers' perceptions of church-based programs to provide depression care for African Americans. J Urban Health 2013;90(4):685–98.

47. Allen AJ, Davey MP, Davey A. Being examples to the flock: The role of church leaders and African American families seeking mental health care services. Contemp Fam Ther 2010;32(2):117–34.

48. Marsh C. The beloved community: how faith shapes social justice from the civil rights movement to today. New York, NY: Basic Books; 2008.

49. Lee-Tauler SY, Eun J, Corbett D, et al. A systematic review of interventions to improve initiation of mental health care among racial-ethnic minority groups. Psychiatr Serv 2018;69(6):628–47.

50. Cook BL, Zuvekas SH, Chen J, et al. Assessing the individual, neighborhood, and policy predictors of disparities in mental health care. Med Care Res Rev 2017; 74(4):404–30.

51. Artiga S, Damico A, Garfield R. Estimates of eligibility for ACA coverage among the uninsured by race and ethnicity. Menlo Park (CA): Kaiser Family Foundation; 2015.

52. Artiga S, Orgera K, Damico A. Changes in health coverage by race and ethnicity since implementation of the ACA, 2013-2017. San Francisco, CA: Kaiser Family Foundation; 2019. Issue Brief.

53. Kim G, Parton JM, DeCoster J, et al. Regional variation of racial disparities in mental health service use among older adults. Gerontologist 2013;53(4): 618–26.

An Anti-Racist Approach to Achieving Mental Health Equity in Clinical Care

Rupinder Kaur Legha, MD[a],*, Jeanne Miranda, PhD[b]

KEYWORDS

• Racism • Antiracism • Implicit bias • Health disparities

KEY POINTS

- Racism is an important determinant of health and health disparities, but few strategies have been proposed to eliminate racial discrimination from clinical care.
- This article proposes a novel antiracist approach to clinical care that takes into account the racism shaping the clinical encounter and historical arc of racial oppression embedded in health care.
- This approach can be implemented into clinical care, may reduce the harm done by racism, and could serve as a template for antiracist service provision in other sectors, such as education and law enforcement.

Racial minorities in the United States experience higher rates of mortality, greater severity and progression of disease, and higher levels of comorbidity and impairment than do their white counterparts. Repeatedly, racism is found as an important determinant of these health inequities.[1,2] Individual discrimination functions as a psychosocial stressor that triggers physiologic, psychological, and behavioral responses, ultimately leading to downstream mental and physical consequences.[3–6] Repeated day-to-day indignities, such as being treated with less respect than others or receiving poorer service at restaurants and stores, accumulate over time, resulting in the more rapid development of coronary heart disease and the birth of babies lower in weight.[7,8] Black infants are 2 to 3 times as likely as their white counterparts to be born prematurely and/or with low birth weights. Because more than half of African American people report discriminatory experiences in multiple sectors of daily life, and more than 70% of Americans harbor implicit biases toward African American people, racism is an important public health concern.[9]

[a] UCLA Center for Health Services and Society, 10920 Wilshire Boulevard, Suite 300, Los Angeles, CA 90024, USA; [b] Department of Psychiatry and Biobehavioral Sciences, UCLA, UCLA's Center for Health Services and Society, 10920 Wilshire Boulevard, Suite 300, Los Angeles, CA 90024, USA
* Corresponding author.
E-mail address: rlegha@mednet.ucla.edu
Twitter: @NoMoreRacismMD (R.K.L.)

Psychiatr Clin N Am 43 (2020) 451–469
https://doi.org/10.1016/j.psc.2020.05.002
0193-953X/20/© 2020 Elsevier Inc. All rights reserved.

However, clinical care interactions, which potentially treat the downstream consequences of racism, also are vulnerable to racial bias. A third of African Americans report experiencing racial discrimination during clinical care with their physicians.[9] Furthermore, multiple studies have shown pro-white implicit bias among physicians, particularly white physicians, and this bias is significantly related to patient-provider interactions, treatment decisions, treatment adherence, and patient health outcomes.[10–12] For example, minorities with the same presenting characteristics and symptoms have been shown to have physicians order less appropriate cardiac procedures than they do for similar white patients.[13] Minorities experience poorer quality of care, decreased access to care, and fewer preventive services. Pain, in particular, is systematically undertreated among black Americans, children and adults alike, relative to white Americans.[14,15]

Health disparities are complex, the outcome of a multitude of factors that function beyond and within medicine. Factors in the former category include the social determinants of health, health insurance coverage, and availability of quality care. Within the realm of health care, strategies to reduce health disparities have focused on increasing diversity in the workforce, training clinicians in cultural competence and implicit bias, and adapting evidence-based treatments to address the health needs of minority communities.[16–18] However, these strategies have not substantially decreased documented health disparities over time, particularly those related to life expectancy, infant mortality, malnutrition, and diabetes.[1,19] Few strategies have been proposed that target racial discrimination in clinical care.[20] This oversight stands in the face of a predominantly white physician workforce and a majority white male medical leadership that does not mirror the diversity of the broader population.[21,22] Its absence is rendered more visible by the medical profession's legacy of racism, including scientific experimentation and exploitation of enslaved individuals and communities of color.[23,24]

Demands for racial equity and justice in health care and other institutions, such as criminal justice and public education, have mounted in recent years.[20,25] Medical students have been particularly vocal about challenging medicine's relative silence about racism and holding academic medical centers accountable for promoting racial justice in their training and clinical care.[26–28] Antiracist efforts have called for more than just the absence of racism; instead, demanding the dismantling of unjust structures that perpetuate racial inequity in clinical care, training, and research and promoting policies that create justice for all.[29,30] Furthermore, teaching the history of discrimination and injustice for minorities has increasingly been implicated as the necessary foundation for deconstructing health inequities created by racist policies.[30] Despite this growing support and the established role of racism in clinical care, antiracist clinical approaches have not been codified. Striving to fill this gap, this article articulates an antiracist approach to clinical care focused on thoughtfully illuminating the racism shaping providers' and patients' lives and clinical interactions, challenging the historical arc of racial oppression embedded in health care, and preventing undue harm by eliminating racial discrimination in the clinical encounter. Recognizing that achieving equity in the clinical encounter is complex and multifactorial, it focuses on racism because it is frequently overlooked, despite its deleterious impact.[31]

This article highlights the legacy of slavery and the African American experience in particular. The authors acknowledge the need to develop similar approaches focused on the experience of American Indian, Alaska Native, First Nation, and other indigenous communities and the legacy of their collective genocide. The authors believe a similar approach can be adapted to consider the needs of their and other racial, sexual, and gender minority communities. As the adverse effects of discriminatory practices, such as the rescinding of Deferred Action for Childhood Arrivals (DACA), police brutality, and legalizing discriminatory practices toward gender and sexual minority members are enacted, the need to curb discriminatory practices in health care becomes more immediate.[32–35] Health care workers face a unique responsibility to develop and implement anti-discriminatory practices. They also have an important opportunity to codify these practices and, it is hoped, pave the way for others, including teachers in the education system and police officers in the law enforcement, to do the same.

In our antiracist approach to medical care, the authors advocate enacting the following practices, which are highlighted in a case example in **Box 1**.

AN ANTIRACIST APPROACH TO CLINICAL CARE
Admit to Being Racist to Become Antiracist: Clinicians Are More Likely to Do Harm When They Deny Their Racial Biases

Racial and ethnic inequalities, including health inequities, are well documented in the United States, originating from colonial America and persisting, even worsening, today. However, racism is infrequently and inadequately cited, taught, or targeted as the root cause of these inequities.[31,36] Its power derives from the denial and obfuscation of its existence; for example, through the practice of racial discrimination while using nonracial language. Policies such as the war on drugs and stereotypical terms such as welfare queen are key examples. Despite disproportionately targeting or being applied to people of color in a harmful or derogatory way (respectively), they are socially acceptable because they avoid using racial slurs and are expressed in ostensibly racially neutral language.[37]

Leading antiracist scholars, including Ibram Kendi,[38] head of American University's Center for Antiracism, have, therefore, argued that confessing to the racism that each person possesses is a first step toward becoming antiracist. Because racism begins not with the prejudice of individuals but with the policies of political and economic power, Kendi[38] argues that the word racist should be treated as a plain, descriptive term for policies and ideas that create or justify racial inequities, not a personal attack. People are racist when endorsing or supporting racist ideas and policies, and, conversely, they are antiracist when endorsing ideas and policies that promote racial equity. "Not racist," the descriptor that many Americans instinctively adopt, is not the opposite of racist because it claims false neutrality that serves as a mask for racism. Everyone, every day, through action or inaction, speech or silence, is choosing in each moment to be racist or antiracist. Frequently, people are both. Racist as a pejorative accusation that singles out individuals only ensnares people in racism's trap and freezes them in inaction.[38]

Racism pervades multiple systems in the form of housing segregation, educational achievement gaps, as well as health disparities.[36] Health care workers possess power and authority in the clinical encounter, and their patients, by contrast, are vulnerable and dependent on them. For this reason, they are uniquely charged with the responsibility of deliberately acknowledging and owning bias to avoid doing harm. An antiracist approach to clinical care proposes that every clinical interaction be considered either racist or antiracist, perpetuating racism in clinical care or championing against it. Thus, antiracism becomes the guiding framework for all interactions, and identifying and acknowledging racism becomes an opportunity to challenge it with an antiracist clinical intervention. This opportunity is missed when racism is denied, such as by suggesting that socioeconomics matter more; or when defensive emotions, such as anger, guilt, and helplessness, reinstate the racial equilibrium

Box 1
Case study: antiracist approach to clinical care

A 14-year-old female child, self-identifying as black, is brought to a psychiatric emergency room by police in handcuffs after her mother calls 911. The child tried to overdose on her antipsychotic medications, and her mother physically restrained her to stop her. She arrives in the emergency room moving uncomfortably in the restraints, and staff request IM medication

Admit to being racist so as to become antiracist: clinicians are more likely to do harm when they deny their racial biases	Conscious of her own racial background, the child psychiatrist recognizes the risk for advancing discriminatory behavior in the clinical encounter and instead deliberates regarding how to comfort and treat the child in an antiracist manner. She gently communicates that cuffing her was coercive and wrong: "I am so sorry that happened to you when you were suffering and needing help. We want to help you here, not harm you or make you feel worse"
Slow down: pause, heighten racial consciousness, and challenge racism	When staff request IM medication, the clinician refuses and instead pauses to do a brief chart review while considering how racism is operating in the child's life and could enter the clinical encounter; eg, by giving IM medication, failing to mitigate harm, or missing an opportunity to render treatment. She notes previous diagnoses of attention-deficit/hyperactivity disorder and oppositional defiant disorder and a history of behavioral challenges at school
Name and identify racism to challenge it: diagnosis determines treatment	The psychiatrist inquires whether her teachers are white or black and whether she ever feels singled out. The child immediately says that all of her teachers are white, that she is the only black child in her special education classes, and she often feels targeted as "the bad kid." After the child reports still feeling suicidal, the child psychiatrist contacts her mother to discuss hospitalization. The mother adds that the child, who has repeatedly been suspended for behavioral challenges, has been seeing a primary care physician for medication because no child psychiatrists in the area accept her insurance. The child psychiatrist discusses with the mother the risk of children of color being disproportionately punished and funneled into the school-to-prison pipeline
Learn the legacy of racism in American medicine to avoid perpetuating it	The child psychiatrist writes a school letter clarifying diagnosis and recommending supportive, rather than punitive, interventions. The antipsychotic prescribed for agitation is stopped, and an antidepressant is started. These therapeutic interventions are directed at the legacies of communities of color not receiving medical care, as well as

	organized psychiatry's not challenging racism and advancing clinical and research practices reinforcing ideologies of black criminality and violence
First, do no harm: prevent the toxic exposure of racism in the clinical encounter	During team rounds, the psychiatrist discusses the child's history of being harshly disciplined for distress and recommends therapeutic interventions that avoid force and encourage verbalization instead. She calls the mother regularly to assist with barriers in accessing care and to foster collaboration. During the monthly physician meeting, she discusses the police's practice of unnecessarily handcuffing children, explains why doing so can be racist, and elicits strategies to decrease this practice and to standardize other antiracist clinical practices
Abbreviation: IM, intramuscular.	

and prevent meaningful dialogue. Racism is everywhere, rather than nowhere, and clinical care interactions become an opportunity to dismantle, breaking through the wall of silence in health care and beyond.[36,38,39]

Slow Down: Pause to Heighten Racial Consciousness and Prepare for Challenging Racism

Psychologist Daniel Kahneman's[40] work describing how people think both fast and slow is a helpful lens for helping clinicians focus and translate knowledge of racism at the structural level into direct antiracist clinical action during the patient encounter. The fast, automatic brain, governing 95% to 97% of behaviors through the mesolimbic pathway, works from unconscious associations and beliefs. The slow, more deliberate and thoughtful brain, associated with the prefrontal cortex, is activated far less frequently. Even if, in slow thinking, people work to avoid discrimination, it can easily creep into fast thinking. Snap judgments rely on all the associations people have derived, from fictional television shows to news reports. Stereotypes, both the accurate and the inaccurate, exist, both those people would want to use and ones they find repulsive. Implicit or unconscious bias reflects both human nature and socialization. It lives deep within people's brains, governing almost everything they do. Developing an understanding of the power of implicit bias enables people to develop practices to minimize the impact of their unconscious tendencies to categorize, generalize, stereotype, and discriminate. Pausing long enough to heighten racial consciousness can challenge clinicians' implicit biases, thereby curbing discriminatory behavior, and instead positioning them to dismantle the racism shaping the patient experience.[40] Subsequent steps provide practical tools to thoughtfully and deliberately enact an antiracist approach.

Name and Identify Racism First to Challenge it: Diagnosis Determines Treatment

Having consciously rejected the denial of racism, reframed all clinical actions as racist or antiracist, and cemented a foundation of slowed, reflective thinking, naming and identifying racism in clinical care is the next step toward constructing an antiracist approach. With shared language and clearer understanding of how institutions and systems are producing unjust and inequitable outcomes, antiracist clinicians are better equipped to work for change. Countless scholars have emphasized naming and identifying racism as a key step toward dismantling it, bearing in mind that most people do not consciously identify as having racist behaviors or acknowledge their implicit biases, and much racism is disguised.[38,41,42] Shared language and clear vision regarding how individuals, institutions, and systems are producing unjust and inequitable outcomes equip antiracist clinicians to work for change.[43] Kendi[38] specifically says, "The only way to undo racism is to consistently identify and describe it—and then dismantle it." In addition, the diagnosis, the proper identification of racism, then determines the treatment of combating it.

Racism has been defined in a multitude of different terms, and the lack of consensus regarding a clear definition speaks to the failure to mount a meaningful national dialogue regarding racism, to implement a core educational strategy for eliminating racial bias, and to materialize a truth and reconciliation process to redress human rights atrocities committed during slavery and the American Indian genocide.[43] Despite this, a multilevel framework that captures internalized, interpersonally mediated, and institutionalized/structural elements to define racism are most frequently cited, Camara Jones'[42] framework being the best example.[41,42] Many definitions of racism also emphasize its historical origins, noting that race is an artificial construct, rooted in and used to justify and legalize slavery, and constructed on the foundation of white supremacy.[36,43]

Table 1 provides definitions and examples of racism using a multilevel framework.[31,42]

Because almost all interracial encounters are prone to microaggressions, this kind of racism is particularly important to integrating an antiracist approach to clinical care.[41] Microaggressions specific to clinical care have been linked to poorer physical health and health service use[44,45] One paradigm emphasizing the harm experienced by the victim, rather than the act committed by the aggressor, argues that clinical microaggressions can undermine physician-patient relationships, preclude relationships of trust, and therefore compromise the kind and quality of care patients deserve.[46]

Ibram Kendi's[38] work complicates the typical 3-tier multilevel frameworks of racism by emphasizing the racist policies and ideologies that provide the breeding ground for the various levels of racism. Linking racist policy and interpersonal racism, he argues that "racial discrimination is an immediate manifestation of an underlying racial policy. When someone discriminates against a person in a racial group, they are carrying out a policy or taking advantage of the lack of a protective policy."[38] Racial policy, in turn, is sustained by a racist ideology. "The only thing wrong with black people is that we think there is something wrong with black people,"[37] a summative statement Kendi emphasizes repeatedly.

Therefore, although clinicians should be directly attuned to the risk of committing racial microaggressions (the racism most explicitly manifested at the interpersonal level), they should also be conscious of potentially advancing the racism operating at the policy, ideological, and individual levels during the clinical encounter. Racism operating at one level reinforces and derives from racism operating at other levels. Policies that create a 2-tiered system of health care through private versus publicly funded systems of care, with racial minorities over-represented within the public system, are important to consider. Clinicians are in key roles to advocate for antiracist policies for insuring more equitable care.[47] By identifying the policies and ideologies shaping patient experience, diagnosis, treatment, and care, antiracist clinicians are better equipped to traverse racial bias, render just and high-quality care, and to even advocate against structural racism. Coercive clinical practices and diagnosis provide 2 key examples.

Table 1
Types, definitions, and examples of racism

Types of Racism	Definition	Examples
Individual/ internalized	A systemic oppression in reaction to racism whereby people of color internalize the racism that victimizes them. It can lead to conflict among and between people of color	• Low self-esteem • Colorism (stratification by skin tone within communities of color) • Self-hatred and self-devaluation • Stereotyping people of color • Having a sense of inferiority
Interpersonal/ microaggression	General: the brief and common daily verbal, behavioral, or environmental indignities, whether intentional or unintentional, that communicate hostile, derogatory, or negative racial slights and insults toward people of color Clinical taxonomy	• Microassault: an explicit racial derogation meant to hurt the intended victim through name calling, avoidant behavior, or purposeful discriminatory actions • Microinsult: verbal, nonverbal, and environmental communications that subtly convey rudeness and insensitivity that demean a person's racial heritage (eg, asking persons of color how they got their job, suggesting affirmative action) • Microinvalidation: communications that subtly exclude, negate, or nullify the thoughts, feelings, or reality of a person of color (eg, asking people where they are from or were born) • Epistemic microaggressions: intentional/unintentional slights conveyed in speech or gesture by health care providers that dismiss, ignore, ridicule, or otherwise fail to give uptake to claims made by physicians • Emotional microaggressions: physicians and other health care providers fail to take patients' emotional reactions to and experiences of their diagnoses and illnesses seriously • Self-identity microaggressions: health care providers intentionally or unintentionally undermine or do not give uptake to the existential consequences that often accompany experiences of illness
Structural	The totality of ways in which societies foster racial discrimination through mutually reinforcing systems of housing, education, employment, earnings, benefits, credits, health care, and criminal justice	• Residential segregation, in particular, is associated with adverse birth outcomes, increased exposure to air pollutants, decreased longevity, increased risk of chronic disease, and increased rates of homicides. It is also associated with decreased access to quality health care

(continued on next page)

Table 1
(continued)

Types of Racism	Definition	Examples
Policy	Any measure that produces or sustains racial inequity between racial groups; policy defined as written and unwritten law, rules, procedures, processes, regulations, and guidelines that govern people	• Slavery and Jim Crow • Voter suppression • Policy brutality/mass incarceration • School-to-prison pipeline/pushout • Housing segregation/redlining
Ideology	Any idea that suggests one racial group is superior or inferior to another group in any way	• Black criminality/violence; white innocence • Black female hypersexuality; white female sexual purity • Black anger/violence; white people as saviors or promoters of peace • Black family as a so-called tangle of pathology • Strength/resilience of black people, suggesting they have superhuman abilities to tolerate hardship • Inferiority/ignorance of black people; superiority/intelligence of white people

Coercive clinical practices such as the use of seclusion, restraint, and intramuscular medication administration are typically used depending on clinical assessment of acute risk for violence or danger to others. This assessment, in turn, is based on clinical factors such as the mental status examination, recent medical history, and response to medication. However, noticeably absent from clinical guidelines is a consideration of racism and discrimination.[48,49] An antiracist approach expands this clinical assessment by first acknowledging the high risk of abusing power, actualizing pervasive racist ideologies regarding black violence and criminality, and traumatizing people of color with their injudicious use. It then carefully considers the risk for advancing the disproportionate use of punishment and violence against people of color, a phenomenon well documented in law enforcement (eg, police brutality, overpolicing of black communities, and mass incarceration of communities of color) and school settings (eg, oversuspension and expulsion and the resultant school-to-prison pipeline), with needed care.[50–52] Within this paradigm, a young black man arriving in restraints to an emergency department (perhaps brought in against his will on a legal hold by police), is likely to have been victimized by overpolicing of his local community and should be spared additional force when at all possible. Recalling that all actions are either racist or antiracist, antiracist clinicians instead make the experience as therapeutic and treatment oriented as possible; for example, by outreaching family, explicitly acknowledging the toll of racism preceding the clinical encounter, and verbalizing a commitment to avoid its perpetuation in care.

Diagnosis is another key conduit for discriminatory practices that demands a slowed, more reflective consideration of the insidious influence of racist ideologies and policies that are common throughout systems of care. Children of color are frequently embedded in segregated school systems with poor racial concordance between students and teachers/principals who are predominantly white, and these students often experience standardized testing practices and curricular content that is discriminatory.[37,38] They are subjected to harsh disciplinary measures, less frequently offered mental health treatment of behavioral challenges compared with their white peers, and are more likely to be funneled into the juvenile detention system and prison settings.[51–54] Adultification is a common racist ideology undergirding these practices. Closely intertwined with criminalization, it involves seeing children of color as older, more culpable, and less in need of nurturing and support than their white peers.[52] When assessing their disruptive behaviors, in particular, antiracist clinicians go beyond a cursory examination of symptoms, weighing deliberately the sociopolitical context in which their behaviors emerge. Avoiding overpathologizing or even condemning the child, they instead diagnose the racist structures causing detriment. Similar to exercising caution with coercive clinical practices, they can avoid disproportionately diagnosing conduct disorder and oppositional defiant disorder among children of color.[55] Challenging the adultification these children endure, antiracist clinicians can instead work closely with schools and teachers to provide more supportive and treatment-oriented approaches that nurture and protect their healthy development. Explicitly acknowledging the racism children experience validates and supports parents and families, renders structural racism more visible, and potentially protects against further harm.

Learn the Legacy of Racism in American Medicine (and Beyond) to Avoid Perpetuating It

Identifying the historical origins of inequities is considered a key step to understanding why black people are treated poorly and differently in the health care system.[30,56,57] These historical arcs are complex, interrelated, and not openly acknowledged in medical training and care by organized medicine. However, their identification is the foundation for codifying antiracist clinical practices to challenge them. American medicine was no different from other major American institutions by serving as a vehicle for legitimizing slavery, the backbone of the burgeoning US economy in the nineteenth century. Common medical school pedagogies involved determining whether or not enslaved people were sick or feigning illness and how best to provide treatment of aberrant behavior, which often consisted of disciplinary measures more accurately resembling human rights abuses and torture.[58] Myths about physical racial differences were used to justify slavery, eventually giving rise to the scientific racism that fueled imperialism and colonization in the nineteenth and twentieth centuries.[59]

American psychiatrists pathologized enslaved people who attempted to risk their lives by running away or who refused to work, diagnosing them with illnesses such as drapetomania or dysesthesia aethiopica. The prescribed treatment was whipping. In the 1960s, psychiatrists characterized angry politically active black men involved in the civil rights movement as having a reactive psychosis. Antipsychotic advertisements from that era sometimes featured angry, threatening cartoons of black men. Pathologizing the emotional and behavioral experiences of black people, rather than condemning the racist policies and practices being protested against, reflects a larger pattern of blaming the individual, rather than condemning more macro-level racist policies and practices. It also perpetuated a narrative of racial difference by suggesting a propensity to violence and criminality among black people.[37,60] This legacy lives on; for example, through the overdiagnosis of disruptive behavior disorders among children of color, caused by implicit biases and inadequate consideration of the disproportionate punishing and policing of these children in school settings.[55] Similar concerns might be raised when accusing a patient of color of malingering. Remarkably, during the Jim Crow Era when white people lynched thousands of black people, massively suppressed black voting rights, and willfully denied black people access to health care, organized psychiatry offered no condemnation of the white rage and white supremacy behind it.[37,61,62] Further underscoring organized psychiatry's complicity with racism and white supremacy, this silence was despite the substantial efforts black psychiatrists made to draw attention to racism's far-reaching impact on black mental health.[63,64]

More recently, a study examining biological causes of violence and its link to parenting practices used juvenile detention records to identify the siblings of violent youth and then used the now-banned drug fenfluramine on more than 30 children, all of whom were children of color. Only when family members sought legal support did the study come under scrutiny. Although the associated academic institutions, Columbia and Mount Sinai, were investigated, neither was formally sanctioned. In addition, several preeminent medical publications did not note any concerns regarding the ethics, risk of racism, or public outcry in publishing study findings.[65] The attempt to link violence to individual biology, rather than the larger social forces of poverty, unemployment, and overpolicing, has long been a focal point of psychiatry and a conduit for advancing a narrative of racial difference and the ideology of black criminality.[23,24]

These examples draw attention to (but do not fully describe) the racism embedded in American medicine and the key role that justifying slavery played in the growth of the medical profession in the nineteenth century.[66–68] Nonetheless, they articulate key trajectories regarding the legacy of slavery in the profession (highlighted in **Table 2**) and provide insight into how racial bias originated in health care. Antiracist clinicians consciously articulate how American medicine and psychiatry were no different from other major American institutions (economic, educational, legal, housing,

Table 2
Legacy of racism in health care directed against African American people

Examples of Arcs	Historical Examples	Contemporary Manifestations
Physical exploitation and human rights abuses	• Scientific experimentation on enslaved people (alive and deceased); perfecting experimental surgeries (eg, cesarean section and ovariotomy) on enslaved women before performing them on all women • Medical school pedagogies focused on maximizing labor and reproductive capacity of enslaved people • Forced sterilization programs, including unnecessary hysterectomies as practice for medical students or as part of eugenics programs (so-called Mississippi appendectomies)	• Coercive clinical practices directed at people of color (disproportionate reporting of cases to child protective services; overdiagnosis of schizophrenia; excessive use of restraints) • Fenfluramine study on children examining link between biology, parenting, and aggression
Narrative of racial difference	• Medical forefathers such as Benjamin Rush (so-called father of American Psychiatry) laid racial inferiority foundations, categorizing black people as subhuman, different from white people, and biologically inferior • Leading psychiatrists pathologizing resistance to slavery • Experimentation on enslaved people justified by belief that they are biologically different (eg, more resistant to pain) • Scientific racism and the pseudoscience of racial difference based on unscientific, descriptive practices, such as phrenology, craniotomy	• Medical students still believe black people experience less pain • Diagnostic frameworks/fallacies for people of color (overdiagnosis of schizophrenia/psychosis and conduct disorders)

(continued on next page)

Table 2
(continued)

Examples of Arcs	Historical Examples	Contemporary Manifestations
Denial and segregation of medical services	• Flexner Report's closure of all but 2 of the 7 historically black medical schools, worsening the physician shortage for black communities • Reconstruction was the nadir of black health status, with staggering death rates among black people caused by poverty and poor housing and sanitation following abolition • Established in 1847, the AMA gained control of hospitals, the medical education system, and professional societies; it supported segregation as its official national policy until 1968	• Racism in health care delivery (not offering treatment to people of color)
White male predominance	• Barring black people from entering medical school during the nineteenth century • AMA allowing local medical societies to ban black physicians until the 1970s	• Crisis of black male physicians (no improvement in >35 y) • Limited number of black faculty • Predominance of white male department chairs
Silence	• AMA did not apologize for barring black professional advancement until 2008 • Organized psychiatry did not speak out regarding fenfluramine study • Some sources estimate that nearly 60% of all enslaved women were sexually assaulted and nearly 1 out of 3 enslaved children were separated from their parents; there has never been any formal acknowledgment of this trauma and its aftermath	• No formal plan to address the legacy of racism and slavery in medicine • Lack of commentary regarding reparations for health care • Lack of antiracist medical training • Lack of recognition of the contributions of black people who were experimented on or exploited

Black (physician) activism

- Fannie Lou Hamer's campaign for reproductive justice (forced sterilization, Mississippi appendectomy)
- Ida B. Wells' antilynching campaign
- NAACP pushing for universal health care (1950s)
- Black physicians desegregated major American hospitals in the 1920s
- NMA lobbied the passage of Medicare and Medicaid to make the health system available to black people, the indigent, and the handicapped

- White Coats for Black Lives (Racial Justice Report Card)

Abbreviations: AMA, American Medical Association; NAACP, National Association for the Advancement of Colored People; NMA, National Medical Association.
Data from Refs. [67,68,72]

political) in justifying slavery and failing to condemn Jim Crow violence. This insight facilitates the slower, more reflective thinking needed to challenge the automatic fast thinking resulting in implicit bias. Key strategies for subsequently translating this knowledge into clinical practice include avoiding coercion and abusive practices, reconsidering diagnosis against this historical landscape, and making every effort to provide treatment to ensure there are no missed care opportunities.

First, Do No Harm: Prevent the Toxic Exposure of Racism in the Clinical Encounter

Because of this historical context and the known health consequences of racism, any act of racism, no matter how small, is a toxic exposure for patients and a sentinel event for the health care system. Inadequate or negligent care of minorities who have weathered or even died of racism across generations, particularly within a caregiving profession that violated its most basic oath, constitutes grave medical error. Accordingly, the risk of racism should always be acknowledged and accounted for by clinicians as if it were a vital sign. This consideration is particularly relevant, given the significant power differentials between clinicians and patients and the risk of the former using power to enact racial subordination of the latter.

Within this framework, good intentions are irrelevant, rather it is the impact of racism (particularly the health consequences) that defines the focus.[69] Clinicians operationalize an antiracist approach to clinical care by reviewing the definitions of racism (see **Table 1**) to see where they might be operating in the patient's experience and by checking for touchpoints and direct links to the historical arcs of racism characterizing medicine and health care more broadly (see **Table 2**). The overarching goal is to protect patients of color against the daily assault of racism embedded in the health care system, and, whenever possible, beyond. The process is deliberate and thoughtful to ensure clinicians do not default to the fast, automatic thinking behind racist implicit biases. The moments when a lead clinician argues that something has nothing to do with race (or racism) or responds with silence if the role of racism is raised are precisely the moments when an antiracist approach to clinical care should be actualized.

Incorporating antiracist dialogue into the clinical encounter traverses the wall of silence characterizing organized medicine's stance on issues of justice and disrupts the legacy of racism in health care. Faculty who benefit from white supremacy bear a greater responsibility for illuminating the invisible forces of racism that shape patients' experiences. Faculty and trainees of color, who face disproportionate professional and personal burdens because of racism and discrimination, should not solely be tasked with improving the system.[70] Case discussions, team treatment planning, grand rounds, didactics, and other treatment and educational opportunities should become the vehicle for these conversations.

LIMITATIONS AND NEXT STEPS

This article describes an antiracist approach to clinical care focused on elucidating the racism shaping providers' and patients' lives and clinical interactions, reversing the historical arc of racial oppression embedded in the health care system, and preventing the toxic exposure to racism in the clinical encounter. Although this approach's ultimate goal is to eliminate health inequities, the authors fully acknowledge their complexity and rooting in structural racism and social determinants of health, which cannot be overcome in a single clinical encounter.[27,29,50] Nonetheless, this approach responds to the burgeoning emphasis on addressing implicit bias and promoting racial justice in health care. It joins other recent antiracist curricular materials developed to challenge racism in health care. Furthermore, it can be implemented immediately by clinicians, can potentially reduce harm experienced by patients, and could facilitate more systemic change in the future by shifting culture and promoting meaningful racial dialogue now.[71]

More data regarding the most common acts of racism taking place in mental health care are needed; however, measuring and tracking (ie, diagnosing) these clinical microaggressions is complex. Family separation has disproportionately affected families of color through slavery, forced relocations, and more recently through mass incarceration. Given these findings, what does it mean when clinicians alienate or antagonize parents of color, are unable or unwilling to partner with them, or disproportionately report them to family services? Are clinicians intervening clinically on the patient's behalf or doing more harm by subscribing to racist ideologies regarding inadequate parenting or pathologic families? Given the legacy of segregating and denying health care services to people of color, what are the implications of fast-tracking out of care a person of color with a documented mental health history seeking shelter but with no acute psychiatric emergency? What does it mean for health care providers to prescribe antipsychotic medications to an agitated child in foster care with an established trauma history whose parents are not available to advocate for the child? How does the overrepresentation of children of color in foster and juvenile justice settings govern antiracist approaches to their care?

Racial disparities permeating the economy, housing, education, and the law raise serious concerns regarding whether certain clinical practices, although potentially justified by a current clinical presentation, do more harm than good to people of color in the long term. Although clarifying answers to these complex questions might take time, initiating dialogue among clinicians, particularly given that the mental health workforce does not mirror the racial diversity of the US population, is an important and immediate next step in leveraging an antiracist approach. Remaining silent or denying the presence of racism in clinical care not only stands in the face of growing demands for antiracist health care but it also perpetuates a legacy of racial injustice that demands to be challenged.

DISCLOSURE

Drs R.K. Legha and J. Miranda have no financial interests or potential conflicts of interest to report.

REFERENCES

1. Agency for Healthcare Research and Quality. 2018 National healthcare quality and disparities report. Rockville (MD): U.S. Department of Health and Human Services; 2019.

2. Institute of Medicine of the National Academies. How far have we come in reducing health disparities? Washington, DC: The National Academies Press; 2012.

3. Lewis T, Cogburn C, Williams D. Self-reported experiences of discrimination and health: scientific advances, ongoing controversies, and emerging issues. Annu Rev Clin Psychol 2015;11:407–40.

4. Paradies Y, Ben J, Denson N, et al. Racism as a determinant of health: a systematic review and meta-analysis. PLoS One 2015;10:e0138511.

5. Dolezsar CM, McGrath JJ, Herzig AJM, et al. Perceived racial discrimination and hypertension: a comprehensive systematic review. Health Psychol 2014;33:20–34.

6. Williams DR, Mohammed SA. Racism and health I: pathways and scientific evidence. Am Behav Sci 2013;57:1152–73.
7. Black LL, Johnson R, VanHoose L. The relationship between perceived racism/discrimination and health among black american women: a review of the literature from 2003 to 2013. J Racial Ethn Health Disparities 2015;2:11–20.
8. Ferdinand KC, Nasser SA. Disparate cardiovascular disease rates in african-americans: the role of stress related to self-reported racial discrimination. Mayo Clin Proc 2017;92:689–92.
9. Blendon RJ, Miller C, Gudenkauf A, et al. Discrimination in America: experiences and views of African Americans 2017. Available at: https://www.npr.org/assets/img/2017/10/23/discriminationpoll-african-americans.pdf.
10. Fitzgerald C, Hurst S. Implicit bias in healthcare professionals: a systematic review. BMC Med Ethics 2017;18:19.
11. Hall WJ, Chapman MV, Lee KM, et al. Implicit racial/ethnic bias among health care professionals and its influence on health care outcomes: a systematic review. Am J Public Health 2015;105:e60–76.
12. Chapman EN, Kaatz A, Carnes M. Physicians and implicit bias: how doctors may unwittingly perpetuate health care disparities. J Gen Intern Med 2013;28:1504–10.
13. Groeneveld PW, Heidenreich PA, Garber AM. Racial disparity in cardiac procedures and mortality among long-term survivors of cardiac arrest. Circulation 2003;108:286–91.
14. Institute of Medicine. Unequal treatment: confronting racial and ethnic disparities in health care. Washington, DC: The National Academies Press; 2003.
15. Hoffman KM, Trawalter S, Axt JR, et al. Racial bias in pain assessment and treatment recommendations, and false beliefs about biological differences between blacks and whites. Proc Natl Acad Sci U S A 2016;113:4296–301.
16. Purnell TS, Calhoun EA, Golden SH, et al. Achieving health equity: closing the gaps in health care disparities, interventions, and research. Health Aff 2016;35:1410–5.
17. Williams DR, Costa MV, Odunlami AO, et al. Moving upstream: how interventions that address the social determinants of health can improve health and reduce disparities. J Public Health Manag Pract 2008;14(Suppl):8–17.
18. Santiago CD, Miranda J. Progress in improving mental health services for racial-ethnic minority groups: a ten-year perspective. Psychiatr Serv 2014;65:180–5.
19. National Academy of Sciences Engineering and Medicine. Communities in action: pathways to health equity. Washington, DC: National Academies Press; 2017.
20. Hardeman RR, Medina EM, Kozhimannil KB. Structural racism and supporting black lives - the role of health professionals. N Engl J Med 2016;375:2113–5.
21. Laurencin C, Murray M. An American crisis: the lack of black men in medicine. J Racial Ethn Health Disparities 2017;4:317–21.
22. Rodríguez JE, López IA, Campbell KM, et al. The role of historically black college and university medical schools in academic medicine. J Health Care Poor Underserved 2017;28:266–78.
23. Gamble VN. Under the shadow of Tuskegee: African Americans and health care. Am J Public Health 1997;87:1773–8.
24. Washington HA. Medical apartheid: the dark history of medical experimentation on Black Americans from colonial times to the present. New York: Doubleday; 2006.
25. Alexander M. The new Jim crow. New York: The New Press; 2010.

26. Ahmad NJ. The need for anti-racism training in medical school curricula. Acad Med 2017;92:1073.
27. White coats 4 black lives. Racial justice report card. 2018. Available at: http://whitecoats4blacklives.org/wp-content/uploads/2018/04/WC4BL-Racial-J. Accessed January 15, 2020.
28. Acosta D, Ackerman-Barger K. Breaking the silence: time to talk about race and racism. Acad Med 2017;92:285–8.
29. Bassett MT. #blacklivesmatter-a challenge to the medical and public health communities. N Engl J Med 2015;372:1085–7.
30. The National Academics of Sciences Engineering and Medicine. Framing the dialogue on race and ethnicity to advance health equity: proceedings of a workshop. Washington, DC: The National Academies Press; 2016.
31. Bailey ZD, Krieger N, Agénor M, et al. Structural racism and health inequities in the USA: evidence and interventions. Lancet 2017;389:1453–63.
32. Venkataramani AS, Tsai AC. Dreams deferred — the public health consequences of rescinding DACA. N Engl J Med 2017;377:1707–9.
33. Alang S, McAlpine D, McCreedy E, et al. Police brutality and black health: setting the agenda for public health scholars. Am J Public Health 2017;107:662–5.
34. Raifman J, Moscoe E, Austin SB, et al. Association of state laws permitting denial of services to same-sex couples with mental distress in sexual minority adults: a difference-in-difference-in-differences analysis. JAMA Psychiatry 2018;75:671–7.
35. Gostin LO, Friedman EA, Wetter SA. Responding to COVID-19: how to navigate a public health emergency legally and ethically. Hastings Cent Rep 2020;50:1–5.
36. Hayes-Greene D, Love BP. The groundwater approach. The Racial Equity Institute; 2018. Available at: https://www.racialequityinstitute.com/groundwaterapproach.
37. Kendi IX. Stamped from the beginning: the definitive history of racist ideas in America. New York: Nation Books; 2016.
38. Kendi I. How to be an antiracist. New York: One World; 2019.
39. DiAngelo RJ. White fragility: why it's so hard for white people to talk about racism. Boston: Beacon Press; 2018.
40. Kahneman D. Thinking fast and slow. New York: Farrar, Straus and Giroux; 2011.
41. Sue DW, Capodilupo CM, Torino GC, et al. Racial microaggressions in everyday life: implications for clinical practice. Am Psychol 2007;62:271–86.
42. Jones CP. Levels of racism: a theoretic framework and a gardener's tale. Am J Public Health 2000;90:1212–5.
43. May R. Racial equity workshop phase 1: foundations in historical and institutional racism. Greensboro, NC: Racial equity institute; 2019.
44. Gonzales KL, Lambert WE, Fu R, et al. Perceived racial discrimination in health care, completion of standard diabetes services, and diabetes control among a sample of American Indian women. Diabetes Educ 2014;40:747–55.
45. Walls ML, Gonzalez J, Gladney T, et al. Unconscious biases: racial microaggressions in American Indian health care. J Am Board Fam Med 2015;28:231–9.
46. Freeman L, Stewart H. Microaggressions in clinical medicine. Kennedy Inst Ethics J 2018;28:411–49.
47. Miranda J, Snowden LR, Legha RK. Policy effects on mental health status and mental health care disparities. In: Goldman H, Frank R, Morrissey JP, editors. The Palgrave handbook of American mental health policy. Cham, Switzerland: Springer International Publishing; 2020. p. 331–64.
48. Garriga M, Pacchiarotti I, Kasper S, et al. Assessment and management of agitation in psychiatry: expert consensus. World J Biol Psychiatry 2016;17:86–128.

49. Gerson R, Malas N, Feuer V, et al. Best practices for evaluation and treatment of agitated children and adolescents in the emergency department: consensus statement of the american association for emergency psychiatry. West J Emerg Med 2019;20:409–18.

50. García JJL, Sharif MZ. Black lives matter: a commentary on racism and public health. Am J Public Health 2015;105:e27–30.

51. Crenshaw K, Ocean P, Nanda J, et al. Black girls matter: pushed out, overpoliced and underprotected. New York: African American Policy Forum; 2014.

52. Epstein R, Blake JJ, Gonzalez T. Girlhood interrupted: the erasure of black girls' childhood. Washington, DC: Georgetown Law Center on Poverty and Inequality; 2017.

53. Wald J, Losen DJ. Defining and redirecting a school-to-prison pipeline. New Dir Youth Dev 2003;2003:9–15.

54. Abramovitz R, Mingus J. Unpacking racism, poverty, and trauma's impact on the school-to-prison pipeline. In: Carten A, Siskind A, Greene M, editors. Strategies for deconstructing racism in the health and human services. New York: Oxford University Press; 2016. p. 245–65.

55. Fadus MC, Ginsburg KR, Sobowale K, et al. Unconscious bias and the diagnosis of disruptive behavior disorders and ADHD in African American and Hispanic youth. Acad Psychiatry 2020;95–102. https://doi.org/10.1007/s40596-019-01127-6.

56. Coates TN. The case for reparations. Magazine article; 2014. Available at: https://doi.org/10.1177/004057366902600305.

57. Williams DR, Collins C. Reparations: a viable strategy to address the enigma of African American health. Am Behav Sci 2004;47:977–1000.

58. Willoughby C. Pedagogies of the black Body: race and medical education in the antebellum United States. New Orleans, LA: Tulane University Digital Library; 2016.

59. Roberts DE. Fatal invention: how science, politics, and big business re-create race in the twenty-first century. New York: New Press; 2011.

60. Myers D. Drapetomania: rebellion, defiance and free black insanity in the antebellum United States. Los Angeles, CA: UCLA; 2014.

61. Anderson C. White rage: the unspoken truth of our racial divide. New York: Bloomsbury; 2016.

62. Lynching in America: confronting the legacy of racial terror. Equal Justice initiative. Available at: https://eji.org/reports/lynching-in-america. Accessed June 7, 2019.

63. Gordon-Achebe K, Hairston DR, Miller S, et al. Origins of racism in American medicine and psychiatry. In: Medlock M, Shtasel D, Trinh N-H, et al, editors. Racism and psychiatry: contemporary issues and interventions. Champagne (France): Springer; 2019. p. 3–19.

64. Comer JP, Hill H. Social policy and the mental health of black children. J Am Acad Child Psychiatry 1985;24:175–81.

65. Shamoo AE, Tauer CA. Ethically questionable research with children: the fenfluramine study. Account Res 2002;9:143–66.

66. Starr P. The social transformation of American medicine. New York: Basic Books; 1982.

67. Byrd WM, Clayton LA, Ebrary I. A medical history of African Americans and the problem of race, beginnings to 1900. New York: Routledge; 2000.

68. Byrd WM, Clayton LA. An American health dilemma: a history of blacks in the health system. J Natl Med Assoc 1992;84:189–200.

69. Williams DR, Lawrence JA, Davis BA. Racism and health: evidence and needed research. Annu Rev Public Health 2019;40:105–25.
70. Cyrus KD. medical education and the minority tax. J Am Med Assoc 2017;317: 1833–4.
71. Sue DW, Lin AI, Torino GC, et al. Racial microaggressions and difficult dialogues on race in the classroom. Cultur Divers Ethnic Minor Psychol 2009;15:183–90.
72. Prather C, Fuller TR, Jeffries WL, et al. Racism, african american women, and their sexual and reproductive health: a review of historical and contemporary evidence and implications for health equity. Health Equity 2018;2:249–59.

Achieving Mental Health Equity: Children and Adolescents

Toi Blakley Harris, MD[a,b,c], Sade C. Udoetuk, MD[d],
Sala Webb, MD, CPH[e], Andria Tatem, MD[f],
Lauren M. Nutile, MD, MS[g], Cheryl S. Al-Mateen, MD[h,i],*

KEYWORDS

- Mental health disparities • Child mental health interventions • Mental health equity
- Pediatric mental health • Child and adolescent population

KEY POINTS

- Providing education to providers about the cultures that they are treating will assist with a community's participation in mental health care.
- Integrated care between pediatric/primary care providers and psychiatric services can strengthen access to mental health care.
- Hiring multicultural staff members can help to mitigate cultural disparities in mental health care.

[a] Psychiatry, Institutional Diversity, Inclusion and Equity & Student and Trainee Services, Center of Excellence in Health Equity, Training and Research, PI/PD, Baylor College of Medicine, 1 Baylor Plaza, Houston, TX 77030, USA; [b] Pediatrics, Institutional Diversity, Inclusion and Equity & Student and Trainee Services, Center of Excellence in Health Equity, Training and Research, PI/PD, Baylor College of Medicine, 1 Baylor Plaza, Houston, TX 77030, USA; [c] Family and Community Medicine, Institutional Diversity, Inclusion and Equity & Student and Trainee Services, Center of Excellence in Health Equity, Training and Research, PI/PD, Baylor College of Medicine, 1 Baylor Plaza, Houston, TX 77030, USA; [d] Menninger Department of Psychiatry and Behavioral Sciences, Baylor College of Medicine, One Baylor Plaza, MS Stop 350, Houston, TX 77030, USA; [e] Behavioral Health, Comprehensive Medical & Dental Plan, Arizona Department of Child Safety, 3003 North Central Avenue, Phoenix, AZ 85012, USA; [f] Department of Pediatrics, Baylor College of Medicine/Texas Children's Hospital, 6701 Fannin Street, Suite 1540, Houston, TX 77030, USA; [g] Department of Psychiatry, Virginia Treatment Center for Children, PO Box 980489, Richmond, VA 23298-0489, USA; [h] Department of Psychiatry, Virginia Treatment Center for Children, Virginia Commonwealth University, PO Box 980489, Richmond, VA 23298-0489, USA; [i] Department of Pediatrics, Virginia Treatment Center for Children, Virginia Commonwealth University, Richmond, VA, USA
* Corresponding author.
E-mail address: Cheryl.Al-Mateen@vcuhealth.org
Twitter: doc2be2014 (A.T.)

Psychiatr Clin N Am 43 (2020) 471–485
https://doi.org/10.1016/j.psc.2020.06.001
0193-953X/20/© 2020 Elsevier Inc. All rights reserved.

INTRODUCTION

Researchers have documented that children and adolescents from minority groups may be impacted negatively by social determinants of health (eg, economic stability, neighborhood and physical environment, education, food and community, and social context) at rates that are disproportionate to their peers (**Fig. 1**).[1] Although there have been improvements with reductions in infant mortality rates across all mothers, African American, black Latinx, and American Indian/Alaskan Native women have rates that are significantly higher than white, Asian, and white Latinx women.[2] Health status has continued to be impacted by age, gender, race, ethnicity, and insurance status.[3] For example, African American, American Indian/Alaska Native, and Latinx respondents to a study endorsed an increased rate of poor health in comparison with their Asian and white counterparts.[1,4,5] Mental health inequities in child, adolescent, and transitional youth populations have also been documented. Those populations with a disproportionate level of risk factors related to poverty, food insecurity, exposure to violence, and/or repeated exposure to discrimination and racism have an increased risk of the following disorders: depression, trauma-related disorders, aggressive and disruptive behaviors, anxiety, substance use, and eating disorders. The presence of these disorders may impact employment ability.[1,5–9] Psychiatrists must be aware of the heterogeneity of all racial and ethnic groups in considering these factors.[10]

Health equity is "the attainment of the highest level of health for all people," and a goal of the US Department of Health and Human Services.[11–13] This article briefly reviews the influences of protective and risk factors of child and adolescent mental health, explores promising practices and outcomes of evidence-based programs designed to improve the mental health of youth, and considers barriers for accessing high-quality child and adolescent mental health service delivery systems. The authors provide recommendations for practice improvements, policy, and funding that will support mental health equity in child and adolescent populations.

CHILDHOOD EXPERIENCES

The influence of childhood positive and negative experiences on adult functioning and health has been described. In recent years, the scope of Adverse Childhood Experiences (ACEs) was expanded by Burke-Harris and Renschler[14] to include ACEs that disproportionately affect marginalized groups (eg, racism, foster care placement). Individuals who have experienced 4 or more ACEs have 4 to 12 times increased risk for substance use disorder, depression, and suicide attempts, as well as increased risk for smoking, poor self-rated health, sexually transmitted infections, sedentary lifestyle, obesity, heart disease, cancer, chronic lung disease, and liver disease.[15] Youth who are from racial, ethnic, gender, or sexual minority backgrounds,[16–18] and those who are immigrants, poor, or from neighborhoods and family structures that are less optimal, have amplified risk factors. To mitigate against risk factors, researchers continue to examine the protective influence of early childhood experiences identified as Benevolent Childhood Experiences (BCEs) or Counter-ACES.[19] Examples of BCEs include feeling safe with a caregiver, having one good friend, beliefs that provided comfort, good neighbors, and a predictable household routine.[20]

EVIDENCE-BASED CLINICAL SOLUTIONS TO INCREASE MENTAL HEALTH EQUITY FOR YOUTH

Numerous programs and treatments have been implemented to address mental health disorders in children and adolescents. There are fewer data available for evidence-based programs improving mental health in minority children than for majority populations. Although several pilot studies and novel ideas are being tested, the published data in this arena are minimal. **Table 1**[21–23] summarizes evidence-based clinical solutions in the literature emphasizing (1) clinical trials in the United States (2010–present), (2) publications with 10% or greater participation from minority populations, and (3) nonpharmacological interventions for various mental health disorders in youth vetted as evidence-based practices by the Substance Abuse and Mental Health Services Administration (SAMHSA) Resource Center.[34]

Interventions are divided into 3 categories of prevention: primary, secondary, and tertiary, aimed at improving functionality and minimizing the impact of a given disorder. Some interventions use technology to increase access to services or provide psychoeducation that may have previously been unavailable to minority children and families because of structural, social, and cultural barriers.

Primary interventions focus on the social determinants of health and the prevention of psychiatric and substance misuse disorders. Due to the increased risk for disorders and disease progression from social determinants of health, other important areas for intervention at the public health level would include programming that improves factors such as food security, built environments, neighborhood safety, education and health care, intrafamily violence, employment of parents, and social isolation.[35]

The 2019 consensus report from the National Academies of Sciences, Engineering and Medicine, states: "the single most important factor in promoting positive psychosocial, emotional, and behavioral well-being in children is having safe, stable, and nurturing relationships with their mother, father, or other primary caregivers."[36] The Reach Out, Stay Strong, Essentials (ROSE) classes for mothers of newborns or the Mothers and Babies educational programming are evidence-based Healthy Start interventions shown to decrease rates of maternal depression.[37] Home-based visits to families during pregnancy and infancy positively effect parental capacity and enhance child development.[38] Similarly, there is evidence that young children with delayed language acquisition, or from low learning stimulating home environments, are at a higher risk for depression during grade school,[39] emphasizing the need for programs such as Head Start, which provide services to families of preschoolers to promote school readiness. Despite inconsistent findings of sustained benefits to Head Start participation overall, a large randomized controlled study showed that African American and Spanish-speaking children had some improved socio-emotional and cognitive performance through the third grade.[40]

Secondary interventions involve early identification of mental health disorders. Two validated screening tools are used for identifying youth at risk for substance use and suicide, respectively. The Screening to Brief Intervention (S2BI), a screening tool for alcohol, marijuana, and tobacco use in youth has been found to identify high-risk users and provide them with resources in pediatric medical settings.[41] It can be used by a clinician or self-administered. The Ask Suicide Screening Questions (ASQ) Toolkit is a National Institute of Mental Health (NIMH)-created and validated tool that can be administered in any pediatric medical setting and is available in many languages.[42] It identifies youth at high risk for suicide and can help determine whether further intervention and referrals are needed. Because youth spend a significant amount of time in schools, school-based interventions are practical to address mental health needs. Screening interventions and programs that have been described in the literature are summarized in **Table 2**.[41–44]

Tertiary interventions are designed to improve functioning or minimize the impact of mental health disorders. Pharmacotherapy, individual and family psychotherapy, and psychoeducation are examples of tertiary interventions and can produce successful results when the presence of disorders has been established.

Table 1
Examples of evidence-based nonpharmacological interventions

Risk/Condition	% Minority Participants, (N)	Intervention	Results	Study
At risk for child abuse and neglect due to poverty/family instability	90% minority (195)	Triple P Online social media and gaming Smartphone features for parents	Decreased behavioral problems at school and parent-reported stress	Love et al,[21] 2016
At risk for PTSD due to history of sexual trauma	35% minority (158)	Trauma-Focused Cognitive-Behavioral Therapy for children	Reduced PTSD criteria	Mannarino et al,[22] 2014
At risk for alcohol use disorders	100% Mexican American (420)	Bridges/Puentes family-focused workshops for children/teens and families	Reduced alcohol use and binge drinking at 5 y poststudy	Gonzalez et al,[23] 2018
At risk for alcohol, nicotine and marijuana use disorders	100% Native American (107)	Living in 2 Worlds curriculum for children/teens	Reduced cigarette use	Kulis et al,[24] 2017
Risky alcohol drinking behavior	21% minority (836)	Brief Intervention given by therapist or self-administered computer program in ER	Reduced DUIs or alcohol-related injuries	Cunningham et al,[25] 2015
At risk for psychosis	32% minority (166)	Family-Focused Therapy for children and families	Reduced positive and negative symptoms of psychosis	O'Brien et al,[26] 2014
Positive screen for anxiety	52% minority (52)	10 Yoga Ed (yoga poses, guided relaxation, and breathing exercises) sessions before school	Improved emotional and psychosocial quality of life	Bazzano et al,[27] 2018
Conduct disorder diagnosis or family report of behavioral problems	100% black and/or Hispanic (80)	Specialized computer-based individual and family therapy sessions	Decreased conduct symptoms, social aggression, and increased family cohesion	Santisteban et al,[28] 2017
Anxiety disorder	25% minority (96)	Single session of a self-directed web-based learning module for child	Decreased anxiety symptoms at 9-mo follow-up	Schleider & Weisz,[29] 2018

Generalized anxiety disorder, social phobia, separation anxiety	13% minority (92)	Emotion-focused cognitive behavioral therapy for child	Reduced emotional dysregulation	Suveg et al,[30] 2018
Oppositional defiant disorder, conduct disorder	15% minority (81)	Multi-Family group Parent-Child Interaction Therapy	Decreased conduct problems and parent stress. Increased adaptive functioning	Niec et al 2016[31]
Bipolar disorder	48% minority (69)	Child- and Family-Focused Cognitive Behavioral Therapy	Reduced manic and depressive symptoms	West et al,[32] 2014
Major depressive disorder	15% minority (470)	Cognitive Behavioral Therapy or psychoanalytical therapy	Reduced depressive symptoms in both therapy groups	Goodyer et al,[33] 2017

Abbreviations: DUI, driving under the influence; PTSD, posttraumatic stress disorder.
Data from Refs.[21–33]

Table 2
Mental health screening interventions and programs for youth

Tool	Age (y)	Targeted Risk	Setting(s)	Modality	Validated	Author
Screening Brief to Intervention (SB2I)	12–17	Alcohol, marijuana and tobacco use	Primary care	Self- or practitioner-administered online	Yes	Levy et al, 2014[41]
Ask Suicide Screening Questions (ASQ)	10–24	Suicide	ER, primary care, inpatient unit, specialty clinic	Practitioner-administered form	Yes	Horowitz et al,[42] 2012
Ready, Set, Go Review: Screening for Behavioral Health Toolkit	>21	Various emotional and behavioral disorders	School	Administrator-/staff-designed and implemented	No	SAMHSA,[43] 2019
Mental Health First Aid for Youth	12–18	Various emotional and behavioral disorders	Community	Specialized course for anyone interacting with children	No	Gryglewicz et al,[44] 2018

Data from Refs.[41–44]

CLINICIAN-BASED SOLUTIONS TO INCREASE MENTAL HEALTH EQUITY FOR YOUTH

Given that many mental health complaints initially come to light in the office of primary care providers, some researchers have recommended the adoption of an integrated care model[1,45] to provide an interdisciplinary and patient-focused environment for treatment.[46,47] Martinez[47] describes the Nuka system in Alaska as the ultimate example of integrated care, providing the patient with an appointment with 4 people at once for a multidisciplinary approach. The primary care provider, medical assistant, nurse, and coordinator for future care/navigator through the clinic are also trained in local culture and customs and encouraged to get to know their fellow team members to improve interpersonal interactions with the team and patients. In addition, Nuka patients are referred to as customer-owners because they are invested in the health care system by holding advisory roles.[47] This is an example of how increased patient involvement and multidisciplinary appointments are good steps toward providers working together to eliminate disparities in treatment.

Although studies have shown providers' inconsistencies with accurately diagnosing individuals from diverse backgrounds,[48] many clinicians do not recognize the impact of intersectionality of multiple social identities in an individual's clinical presentation and response to treatment. Research has shown that the more ways in which a youth is marginalized (eg, low socioeconomic status, poor education, non-English speaking), the more significant the potential for disadvantage.[49–53] To appreciate the intersectionality within a patient helps a clinician to consider their own biases and understanding of a patient's social identities. Factors such as race, gender, sexuality, religion, abilities, and language may affect a child's perception of and interaction with others. The clinician should also consider power dynamics related to these aspects of the patient's identities by considering ways in which the clinician may occupy a position of privilege in comparison to the patient as well as by avoiding the assumption that being part of the same group as the patient (eg, a black female) means the clinician has a similar experience to the patient.[49,54]

Agencies and individual practices can address the concern of cultural differences by hiring multicultural or multilingual individuals for positions ranging from the front desk staff and team members who schedule patients to direct patient care providers.[1] All mental health team members, including leadership and administration, can expand their knowledge about the populations and cultures being served by the practice. Practices may include the use of paraprofessionals such as community health workers (eg, *promotores*), family navigators, or other support workers to help coordinate access to outside resources and follow-up care.[55]

Screening methods for common disorders like anxiety and depression should be available in appropriate languages, with sensitivity to cultural differences in clinical presentation.[55] Language barriers should never play a role in the provision of treatment; thus, interpreters must be accessible (in person when possible). Federal regulations require that health care organizations provide culturally and linguistically appropriate services (CLAS Standards) by delivering competent language assistance to those with limited and other communication needs at no cost. This clinical requirement includes those who require American Sign Language or other forms of language interpretation.[56,57]

The education of mental health team members is not the only vital part of minimizing mental health care disparities; patient education is also important. Practices with interdisciplinary care can provide education about mental health during outpatient visits. Clinics can also make an impact by reaching out to their communities and offering a range of educational programs. Specifically, focusing on parents and providing them with ways to recognize when problems exist and where to turn for help would be beneficial (See **Fig. 1**)[1,2] In addition, providers may choose to serve as mentors for students/trainees that are members of groups underrepresented in medicine to aid with a smoother transition to future employment in the community.[45]

Advocacy planning is another means through which researchers have recommended that clinicians assist with minimizing mental health care disparities in the United States. Advocacy for reducing neighborhood gun violence, increasing availability of programs such as Head Start, and the rehabilitation of low-income neighborhoods can be the nidus for larger-scale change.[2,40] Finally, individual providers often can choose where to open their clinics. Choosing a building within the heart of the neighborhood, easily accessible by public transportation, with hours that increase the chance working-class families can make appointments, may increase the utilization of these clinic services.[47] If there are financial assistance programs that practices are willing to work with, or if pharmacies are located nearby, patients are more likely to be adherent with treatment.

The American Academy of Child and Adolescent Psychiatry (AACAP) Practice Parameters for Cultural Competence in Child and Adolescent Psychiatry Practice recommends that clinicians follow 13 principles that address many of the barriers that relate to the child, families, and their communities, including identifying and addressing the clinician's own biases (**Box 1**).[58] AACAP also has a Practice Parameter on Gay, Lesbian, or Bisexual Sexual Orientation, Gender Nonconformity, and Gender Discordance in Children and Adolescents. This document highlights the practitioner's role in primary, secondary, and tertiary interventions for these youth who are at high risk for developmental and psychosocial challenges that become clinically significant (**Box 2**). These challenges may occur in the family as well as the community.[59] In May 2019, the US Department of Health and Human Services developed continuing education e-programs to help clinicians improve adherence to CLAS Standards. Programs are available for a variety of health professionals, including those working in mental health.[60]

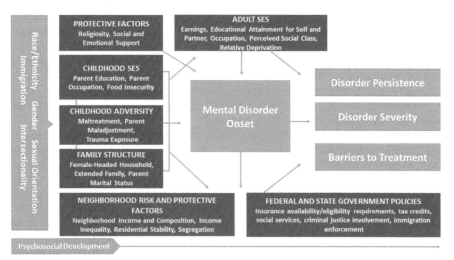

Fig. 1. Conceptual model for child mental health and mental health service disparities. SES, socioeconomic status. (*Adapted from* Alegria M, Green JG, McLaughlin KA, et al. Disparities in child and adolescent mental health and mental health services in the United States. William T. Grant Foundation, New York, New York: 2015; with permission. Available at: https://wtgrantfoundation.org/library/uploads/2015/09/Disparities-in-Child-and-Adolescent-Mental-Health.pdf.)

Box 1
Practice parameters for cultural competence in child and adolescent psychiatric practice

Clinicians should:
1. Identify and address barriers that may prevent obtaining mental health services.
2. Conduct the evaluation in the language in which the child and family are proficient.
3. Understand the impact of dual language competence on the child's adaptation and functioning.
4. Be cognizant of one's own cultural biases and address them.
5. Apply knowledge of cultural differences in development, idioms of distress, and symptomatic presentation to clinical formulation and diagnosis.
6. Assess for history of immigration-related loss or trauma and community trauma and address them in treatment.
7. Evaluate and address acculturation stress and intergenerational acculturation family conflict.
8. Make special effort to include family members and key members of traditional extended families in assessment, treatment planning, and treatment.
9. Evaluate and incorporate the child and family's cultural strengths in treatment interventions.
10. Treat the child and family in familiar settings within their community when possible.
11. Support parents to develop appropriate behavioral management skills compatible with their cultural values and beliefs.
12. Use evidence-based psychological and pharmacologic interventions specific for the child and family's ethnic/racial population.
13. Identify ethnopharmacological factors that may influence the child's response to medications, including side effects.

Data from Pumariega AJ, Rothe E, Mian A, et al. Practice Parameter for Cultural Competence in Child and Adolescent Psychiatric Practice. Journal of the American Academy of Child & Adolescent Psychiatry. 2013;52(10):1101–1115.

SYSTEMIC SOLUTIONS

The literature has provided recommendations to address systemic factors implicated in child and adolescent health inequities that involve defining scope, leveraging existing policies and programs, targeting marketing and education, and increasing stakeholder accountability.

Recommendation 1: Define the Scope

Mental health equity for children and adolescents can mean many things. It conveys that the behavioral and mental health needs of youth should have an equal focus on their physical health needs. It also implies that all youth, regardless of their demographics, should have equal access to quality mental health treatment. Moreover, mental health equity for children and adolescents encompasses the theme that youth mental health should be considered on equal footing with adult mental health. Not only is it easier to devise a plan of action when the problem's components are simplified, it also improves the likelihood of securing potential stakeholder allies needed to advance policy or program improvements.

Recommendation 2: Leverage Existing Policies and Programs

Creating standalone policies on implementing equity in mental health for children and adolescents is not adequate. This isolated approach would have limited value and reach if they are not linked with the programs that address physical health needs and social determinants of health, which may already exist. The Early Periodic

---

Box 2
Principles from the practice parameter on gay, lesbian, or bisexual sexual orientation, gender nonconformity, and gender discordance in children and adolescents

1. A comprehensive diagnostic evaluation should include an age-appropriate assessment of psychosexual development for all youths.

2. The need for confidentiality in the clinical alliance is a special consideration in the assessment of sexual and gender minority youth.

3. Family dynamics pertinent to sexual orientation, gender nonconformity, and gender identity should be explored in the context of the cultural values of the youth, family, and community.

4. Clinicians should inquire about circumstances commonly encountered by youth with sexual and gender minority status that confer increased psychiatric risk.

5. Clinicians should aim to foster health psychosexual development in sexual and gender minority youth and to protect the individual's full capacity for integrated identity formation and adaptive functioning.

6. Clinicians should be aware that there is no evidence that sexual orientation can be altered through therapy, and that attempts to do so may be harmful.

7. Clinicians should be aware of current evidence on the natural course of gender discordance and associated psychopathology in children and adolescents in choosing the treatment goals and modality.

8. Clinicians should be prepared to consult and act as a liaison with schools, community agencies, and other health care providers, advocating for the unique needs of sexual and gender minority youth and their families.

9. Mental health professionals should be aware of community and professional resources relevant to sexual and gender minority youth.

Data from Adelson SL. Practice Parameter on Gay, Lesbian, or Bisexual Sexual Orientation, Gender Nonconformity, and Gender Discordance in Children and Adolescents. Journal of the American Academy of Child & Adolescent Psychiatry. 2012;51(9):957-974.

Screening Detection and Treatment (EPSDT) benefit under Medicaid is one such entity. With EPSDT, Medicaid-eligible children have access to preventive, diagnostic, and treatment services for physical, mental, and dental conditions. The goal of EPSDT "is to assure that all individual children get the health care they need when they need it – the right care to the right child at the right time in the right setting."[61] This sentiment is in complete alignment with ensuring attuned and equitable mental health services for children and adolescents.

There are also opportunities to safeguard that mental health equity is being included within newer initiatives of enhancing mental health services in schools. In 2019, SAMHSA, in conjunction with the Centers for Medicare and Medicaid Services, released official guidance for school and state systems on how to address mental health and substance use issues in schools.[62] Although the document outlined various intervention approaches and funding sources, there was no specific mention of how to culturally tailor these interventions so that they would be most efficacious.

Recommendation 3: Consider Targeted Marketing and Education Approaches

Professionals in the pediatric mental health space should both influence and direct the content of the communications that reach the legislators, administrators, and other health care decision-makers to make youth mental health equity a priority.

Education on the development and maintenance of mental health in childhood and adolescence should be infused throughout the curriculum of medical and health care training institutions to promote this holistic approach to well-being in current and future generations of the health care workforce. Health care providers need to be aware of cultural influences on accessing and using mental health treatment among minority families. Likewise, minority communities may benefit from uniquely tailored mental health promotion and literacy interventions that resonate with their cultural values.[1]

Recommendation 4: Increase Stakeholder Accountability

The current allocation of state and federal funding may leave some health care programs such as the State Children's Health Insurance Program in limbo. Without funding, vulnerable youth will have limited access to mental health services. Historically, the array of mental and behavioral health services for children and adolescents under Medicaid has been rather robust when compared with those covered by commercially available private insurances. To ultimately create mental health equity for the youth in our country, children and adolescents should have equal access to mental health services regardless of the underwriter. In efforts to close these gaps, states and other systems of care have looked to grants from governmental and nongovernmental sources, but these may not be sustainable in the long-term.

One response to that problem has been the creation of accountable care entities. There are many variations on this theme, but one archetype that is supported by the National Academy for State Health Policy promotes having the local community address its health and related needs (such as transportation and housing) by establishing a coalition of community organizations, health systems, and other partners who are not only accountable for controlling costs but improving population health and health equity.[63]

SUMMARY

In this article, risk and protective factors contributing to child and adolescent mental health inequities have been described. The overlapping concepts that contribute to these inequities, including social determinants of health, ACEs, and Counter-ACEs/ Benevolent Childhood Experiences were reviewed. Barriers to receiving care were also explored. When working with diverse populations, clinicians need the capacity to both recognize and appreciate the impact of intersectionality in the clinical setting for accurate diagnoses. Evidence-based evaluation strategies, screening tools, and treatment modalities were summarized.

What lies next? Those who provide or regulate health care must have the vision to realize that establishing a clear priority for mental health equity for children and adolescents is the foundation for our future. Achieving mental health can only come from the systemic recognition that inequity for youth influences mental health for adults, and negatively impacts our society for decades to come.

DISCLOSURE

C.S. Al-Mateen: Book co-editor, chapter co-author for *Cultural Psychiatry in Children Adolescents and Families,* American Psychiatric Publishing (due January 2021); chapter co-author "Diversity and Culture" for *Transition-Age Youth Mental Healthcare,* Springer Publishing (due 2020). Other authors have nothing to disclose.

REFERENCES

1. Alegria M, Vallas M, Pumariega A. Racial and ethnic disparities in pediatric mental health. Child Adolesc Psychiatr Clin N Am 2010;19(4):759–74.
2. Center for Disease Control and Prevention, National Center for Health Statistics United States. Table 2. Infant, neonatal, postneonatal, fetal, and perinatal mortality rates, by detailed race and Hispanic origin of mother - United States, selected years 1983-2017.pdf. 2018. Available at: https://www.cdc.gov/nchs/data/hus/2018/002.pdf. Accessed January 15, 2020.
3. Center for Disease Control and Prevention, National Center for Health Statistics United States. Table 16. Respondent-assessed fair-poor health status, by selected characteristics- United States, selected years 1991-2017.pdf. 2018. Available at: https://www.cdc.gov/nchs/data/hus/2018/016.pdf. Accessed January 15, 2020.
4. Alegría M, Green JG, McLaughlin KA, et al. Disparities in child and adolescent mental health and mental health services in the U.S. New York: A William T. Grant Foundation Inequality Paper. 2015. Available at: https://wtgrantfoundation.org/library/uploads/2015/09/Disparities-in-Child-and-Adolescent-Mental-Health.pdf. Accessed December 26, 2019.
5. Chatterji P, Alegria M, Takeuchi D. Racial/Ethnic differences in the effects of psychiatric disorders on employment. Atlantic Econ J 2009;37(3):243–57.
6. Avenevoli S, Swendsen J, He J-P, et al. Major depression in the national comorbidity survey–adolescent supplement: prevalence, correlates, and treatment. J Am Acad Child Adolesc Psychiatry 2015;54(1):37–44.e2.
7. Aratani Y, Addy S. Disparities in repeat visits to emergency departments among transition-age youths with mental health needs. Psychiatr Serv 2014;65(5):685–8.
8. Merikangas KR, He J, Burstein M, et al. Service utilization for lifetime mental disorders in U.S. adolescents: results of the National Comorbidity Survey–Adolescent Supplement (NCS-A). J Am Acad Child Adolesc Psychiatry 2011;50(1):32–45.
9. Bardach NS, Burkhart Q, Richardson LP, et al. Hospital-based quality measures for pediatric mental health care. Pediatrics 2018;141(6):e20173554.
10. Atdjian S, Vega WA. Disparities in mental health treatment in U.S. racial and ethnic minority groups: implications for psychiatrists. Psychiatr Serv 2005;56(12):1600–2.
11. National Partnership for Action to End Health Disparities. National stakeholder strategy for achieving health equity. U.S. Department of Health and Human Services Office of Minority Health; 2011. p. 233.
12. U.S. Department of Health and Human Services. Mental health: culture, race, and ethnicity—a supplement to mental health: a report of the surgeon general. Rockville (MD): US Department of Health and Human Services, Substance Abuse and Mental Health Services Administration, Center for Mental Health Services; 2001.
13. Bronfenbrenner U. The ecology of human development: experiments by nature and design. Cambridge (MA): Harvard University Press; 1979.
14. Burke Harris N, Renschler T. Center for Youth Wellness ACE-Questionnaire (CYW ACE-Q Child, Teen, Teen SR). Center for Youth Wellness. San Francisco (CA): Center for Youth Wellness; version 7/2015.
15. Felitti V, Anda RF, Nordenberg DF, et al. Relationship of childhood abuse and household dysfunction to many of the leading causes of death in adults – the Adverse Childhood Experiences (ACE) Study. Am J Prev Med 1998;14(4):245–58.

16. Becerra-Culqui TA, Liu Y, Nash R, et al. Mental health of transgender and gender nonconforming youth compared with their peers. Pediatrics 2018;141(5): e20173845.

17. Fergusson DM, Horwood LJ, Beautrais AL. Is sexual orientation related to mental health problems and suicidality in young people? Arch Gen Psychiatry 1999; 56(10):876.

18. Safren SA, Heimberg RG. Depression, hopelessness, suicidality, and related factors in sexual minority and heterosexual adolescents. J Consult Clin Psychol 1999;67(6):859–66.

19. Narayan AJ, Rivera LM, Bernstein RE, et al. Positive childhood experiences predict less psychopathology and stress in pregnant women with childhood adversity: A pilot study of the benevolent childhood experiences (BCEs) scale. Child Abuse Negl 2018;78:19–30.

20. Crandall A, Miller JR, Cheung A, et al. ACEs and counter-ACEs: how positive and negative childhood experiences influence adult health. Child Abuse Negl 2019; 96:104089.

21. Love S, Sanders M, Turner K, et al. Social media and gamification: engaging vulnerable parents in an online evidence-based parenting program. Child Abuse Negl 2016;53:95–107.

22. Mannarino A, Cohen J, Deblinger E, et al. Trauma-focused cognitive-behavioral therapy for children: sustained impact of treatment 6 and 12 months later. Child Maltreat 2012;17(3):231–41.

23. Gonzales NA, Jensen M, Tein JY, et al. Effect of middle school interventions on alcohol misuse and abuse in mexican american high school adolescents: five-year follow-up of a randomized clinical trial. JAMA Psychiatry 2018;75(5):429.

24. Kulis SS, Ayers SL, Harthun ML. Substance use prevention for urban american indian youth: an efficacy trial of the Culturally Adapted Living in 2 Worlds Program. J Prim Prev 2017;38(1–2):137–58.

25. Cunningham R, Chermack S, Ehrlich P, et al. Alcohol interventions among underage drinkers in the ED: a randomized controlled trial. Pediatrics 2015;136(4): e783–93.

26. O'Brien MP, Miklowitz DJ, Candan KA, et al. A randomized trial of family focused therapy with populations at clinical high risk for psychosis: effects on interactional behavior. J Consult Clin Psychol 2014;82(1):90–101.

27. Bazzano A, Anderson C, Hylton C, et al. Effect of mindfulness and yoga on quality of life for elementary school students and teachers: results of a randomized controlled school-based study. Psychol Res Behav Manag 2018;11:81–9.

28. Santisteban D, Czaja S, Nair S, et al. Computer informed and flexible family-based treatment for adolescents: a randomized clinical trial for at-risk racial/ethnic minority adolescents. Behav Ther 2017;48(4):474–89.

29. Schleider J, Weisz J. A single-session growth mindset intervention for adolescent anxiety and depression: 9-month outcomes of a randomized trial. J Child Psychol Psychiatry 2018;59(2):160–70.

30. Suveg C, Jones A, Davis M, et al. Emotion-focused cognitive-behavioral therapy for youth with anxiety disorders: a randomized trial. J Abnorm Child Psychol 2018;46(3):569–80.

31. Niec L, Barnett M, Prewtt M, et al. Group parent-child interaction therapy: a randomized control trial for the treatment of conduct problems in young children. J Consult Clin Psychol 2016;84(8):682–98.

32. West AE, Weinstein SM, Peters AT, et al. Child- and family-focused cognitive-behavioral therapy for pediatric bipolar disorder: a randomized clinical trial. J Am Acad Child Adolesc Psychiatry 2014;53(11):1168–78.e1.

33. Goodyer IM, Reynolds S, Barrett B, et al. Cognitive behavioural therapy and short-term psychoanalytical psychotherapy versus a brief psychosocial intervention in adolescents with unipolar major depressive disorder (IMPACT): a multi-centre, pragmatic, observer-blind, randomised controlled superiority trial. Lancet Psychiatry 2017;4(2):109–19.

34. Substance Abuse and Mental Health Services Administration. Evidence-based practices resource center. Available at: www.samhsa.gov/ebp-resource-center. Accessed January 22, 2020.

35. Shim R, Koplan C, Langheim F, et al. The social determinants of mental health: an overview and call to action. Psychiatric Ann 2014;44(1):22–6.

36. National Academies of Sciences. Engineering, and medicine. Vibrant and Healthy kids: aligning science, practice, and policy to advance health equity. Washington (DC): National Academies Press; 2019.

37. National Institute for Children's Health Quality, Health Resources and Services Administration, U. S. Department of Health and Human Services. Available at: www.healthystartepic.org/resources/evidence-based-practices. Accessed January 22, 2020.

38. Daro D, Klein S, Burkhardt T, et al. Home visiting's impact on parental capacity and child development- measurement options and recommendations. Arlington (VA): James Bell Associates; 2019.

39. Herman KC, Cohen D, Owens S, et al. Language delays and child depressive symptoms: the role of early stimulation in the home. Prev Sci 2016;17(5):533–43.

40. Puma M, Bell S, Cook R, et al. Third grade follow-up to the Head Start impact study: final report. Washington (DC): Office of Planning, Research and Evaluation, Administration for Children and Families, US Department of Health and Human Services; 2012. p. 346.

41. Levy S, Weiss R, Sherritt L, et al. An electronic screen for triaging adolescent substance use by risk levels. JAMA Psychiatry 2014;168(9):822–8.

42. Horowitz L, Bridge J, Teach S, et al. Ask Suicide-Screening Questions (ASQ): a brief instrument for the pediatric emergency department. Arch Pediatr Adolesc Med 2012;166(12):1170–6.

43. Substance Abuse and Mental Health Services Administration. Ready, set, go, review: screening for behavioral health risk in schools. Rockville (MD): Office of the Chief Medical Officer, Substance Abuse and Mental Health Services Administration; 2019.

44. Gryglewicz K, Childs KK, Soderstrom MFP. An evaluation of youth mental health first aid training in school settings. Sch Ment Health 2018;10(1):48–60.

45. Bussing R, Gary FA. Eliminating mental health disparities by 2020: everyone's actions matter. J Am Acad Child Adolesc Psychiatry 2012;51(7):663–6.

46. Sanchez K, Chapa T, Ybarra R, et al. Eliminating health disparities through culturally and linguistically centered integrated health care: consensus statements, recommendations, and key strategies from the field. J Health Care Poor Underserved 2014;25(2):469–77.

47. Martinez ON. Eliminating mental and physical health disparities through culturally and linguistically centered integrated healthcare. J Fam Strengths 2017;17(1):14.

48. Liang J, Matheson BE, Douglas JM. Mental health diagnostic considerations in racial/ethnic minority youth. J Child Fam Stud 2016;25(6):1926–40.

49. Bowleg L. The problem with the phrase women and minorities: intersectionality—an important theoretical framework for public health. Am J Public Health 2012; 102(7):1267–73.
50. Sussman S, Kattari SK, Baezconde-Garbanati L, et al. Commentary: the problems of grouping all adversity into a special populations label. Evaluation & the Health Professions; 2019; 43(1):66-70.
51. Wilson Y, White A, Jefferson A, et al. Intersectionality in clinical medicine: the need for a conceptual framework. Am J Bioeth 2019;19(2):8–19.
52. Betancourt JR. Cross-cultural medical education: conceptual approaches and frameworks for evaluation. Acad Med 2003;78(6):10.
53. Mian AI, Al-Mateen CS, Cerda G. Training child and adolescent psychiatrists to be culturally competent. Child Adolesc Psychiatr Clin N Am 2010;19(4):815–31.
54. American Psychiatric Association. In: Diagnostic and statistical manual of mental disorders, DSM-5. 5th edition. Washington, DC: American Psychiatric Publishing; 2013.
55. Hodgkinson S, Godoy L, Beers LS, et al. Improving mental health access for low-income children and families in the primary care setting. Pediatrics 2017;139(1): e20151175.
56. U.S. Department of Health and Human Services, Office of Minority Health. National CLAS Standards. National Standards for Culturally and Linguistically Appropriate Services (CLAS) in health and health care. 2013. Available at: https://thinkculturalhealth.hhs.gov/assets/pdfs/EnhancedNationalCLASStandards.pdf. Accessed January 12, 2020.
57. Jacobs B, Ryan AM, Henrichs KS, et al. Medical interpreters in outpatient practice. Ann Fam Med 2018;16(1):70–6.
58. Pumariega AJ, Rothe E, Mian A, et al. Practice parameter for cultural competence in child and adolescent psychiatric practice. J Am Acad Child Adolesc Psychiatry 2013;52(10):1101–15.
59. Adelson SL. Practice parameter on gay, lesbian, or bisexual sexual orientation, gender nonconformity, and gender discordance in children and adolescents. J Am Acad Child Adolesc Psychiatry 2012;51(9):957–74.
60. U.S. Department of Health and Human Services Office of Minority Health. Available at: Thinkculturalhealth.hhs.gov/education. Accessed January 22, 2020.
61. Centers for Medicare and Medicaid Services. EPSDT- A guide for states: coverage in the Medicaid benefit for children and adolescents. 2014. Available at: https://www.medicaid.gov/medicaid/benefits/downloads/epsdt_coverage_guide.pdf. Accessed January 22, 2020.
62. Substance Use and Mental Health Services Administration Center for Medicare and Medicaid Services. Guidance to state and school systems on addressing mental health and substance use issues in schools. 2019. Available at: https://store.samhsa.gov/system/files/pep19-school-guide.pdf. Accessed January 22, 2020.
63. National Academy for State Health Policy. Resources for states to address health equity and disparities. 2019. Available at: https://nashp.org/resources-for-states-to-address-health-equity-and-disparities/#toggle-id-2. Accessed January 22, 2020.

Achieving Mental Health Equity: Addictions

Ayana Jordan, MD, PhD[a],*, Myra L. Mathis, MD[b], Jessica Isom, MD, MPH[c,1]

KEYWORDS

- Addiction • Inequity • Treatment • Disparity • Drug policy • Social determinants

KEY POINTS

- Substance use disorders are the number one health problem in the twenty-first century, but only 18% of people receive treatment.
- There are several historical policies related to drug use that have resulted in the systematic exclusion of treatment of minoritized populations experiencing health disparities.
- In the twenty-first century there was a shift from criminalizing substance use to adopting a medical approach, focused on treatment instead of incarceration.
- Equitable addiction treatment should (1) be readily available, (2) attend to multiple needs of an individual, (3) be of adequate duration, and (4) include medications when needed.
- Barriers to treatment include stigma, nonintegrated primary and mental health services, and lack of focus on the social determinants of health.

THE NEED FOR HEALTH EQUITY IN ADDICTION TREATMENT

Despite available treatment options for addiction, there remains an abysmal uptake of treatment initiation and engagement among varying communities. This article carefully examines the existing treatment gap in addiction, drug policies enacted that have contributed to this gap, and the development of the disease model of addiction. The authors also consider how major historical developments explain why certain communities are at higher risk of death and are less likely to engage in care. We then use the opioid crisis to illustrate the existing disparity in addiction treatment among varying communities, highlighting barriers such as institutionalized racism, vulnerabilities in the social determinants of health, and an array of solutions to address these inequities. Finally, we conclude by briefly discussing existing addiction treatment and research models, aimed at minimizing the addiction treatment gap, with

[a] Department of Psychiatry, Yale University School of Medicine, 300 George Street, Suite 901, New Haven, CT 06511, USA; [b] Department of Psychiatry, University of Rochester, 601 Elmwood Avenue, Rochester, NY 14642, USA; [c] Codman Square Health Center, Boston Medical Center, Randolph, Massachusetts, USA
[1] Codman Square Health Center, 637 Washington St, Dorchester, MA 02124
* Corresponding author.
E-mail address: ayana.jordan@yale.edu

Psychiatr Clin N Am 43 (2020) 487–500
https://doi.org/10.1016/j.psc.2020.05.007
0193-953X/20/© 2020 Elsevier Inc. All rights reserved.
psych.theclinics.com

the goal of providing equitable care in urban, suburban, rural, and marginalized communities.

A CONSIDERABLE GAP EXISTS IN ADDICTION TREATMENT

In 2018, approximately 164.8 million Americans aged 12 years or older reported substance use (ie, tobacco, alcohol, or illicit drugs) in the past month, with 20.3 million people meeting criteria for an alcohol or illicit drug use disorder.[1] The impact of unhealthy substance use on the well-being of the US population goes beyond these data alone, as substance use causes more deaths, illnesses, and disabilities than any other preventable health condition.[1] Throughout the late twentieth and early twenty-first century, substance use was identified as the number one health problem in America. Still, many more people need treatment of substance use disorders than are receiving it. In 2018, only 18% of people identified as needing treatment actually received it, leaving 17.5 million people who did not receive care for a treatable health condition.[2]

This treatment gap exists within a unique historical context: with drug policy, addiction treatment models, and health care delivery systems evolving in both independent and intersecting ways. Policy- and systems-based issues have had differential impacts on varying populations, creating stark differences in whom and the environments in which individuals seek treatment of substance use disorders. When considering health inequities in addiction, it is important to give attention to this longitudinal perspective, as it creates a framework for understanding the current treatment landscape.

OVERVIEW: US DRUG POLICY IN THE TWENTIETH CENTURY

The passage of the Harrison Narcotics Tax Act of 1914, regulating the distribution of opium- and coca-containing products, set the tone for drug policy laws of the next century.[3] Initially, a means to tax and register the import, sale, and distribution of opium and coca derivatives, the 1914 law was interpreted as a prohibitive act by law enforcement agencies. In particular, a phrase meant to protect physicians from prosecution when prescribing opioids for health conditions was used to prosecute physicians who prescribed opioids for the treatment of addiction. It was argued that opioid addiction was not a medical condition and, therefore, the use of opioids in such cases was not "in the course of [a physician's] professional practice.[3]" Under this interpretation, some physicians who used morphine to treat heroin addiction were prosecuted and jailed.[4] What resulted from the enforcement of the Harrison Act was a policy landscape that uncoupled addiction from medical practice, leaving drug policy to be fashioned through lenses that stigmatize and criminalize individuals in need of treatment.

As outlined later in **Fig. 1**, many laws regulating the sale and distribution of drugs and alcohol followed, including the National Prohibition Act of 1920, the Marihuana Tax Act of 1937, and the Comprehensive Drug Abuse Prevention and Control Act of 1970.[3] President Nixon declared the "War on Drugs" in the months following the passage of the 1970 law. The drug war was later referred to by one of Nixon's aides as a means to target his political adversaries, namely black people and antiwar activists.[5] President Reagan reignited the War on Drugs in the 1980s, passing the Comprehensive Crime Control Act of 1984 and the Anti-Drug Abuse Acts of 1986 and 1988. Notably, the Anti-Drug Abuse Act of 1986 established 22 new mandatory minimum sentences for drug-related crimes and is responsible for the 100:1 sentencing

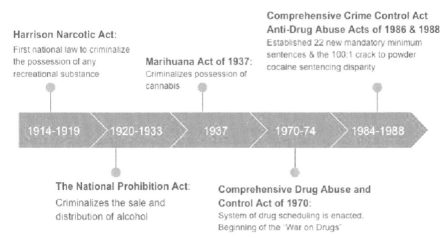

Fig. 1. Timeline of drug policy in the United States.

disparity for crack cocaine versus powder cocaine, which led to disproportionately longer sentences for black people.[3]

The legislative record does not clearly outline any rationale for this dramatic disparity at the time the Anti-Drug Abuse Act of 1986 was passed.[6] It is known, however, that crack cocaine was falsely thought to have more rapid and potent activity in the brain, leading to the erroneous assumption that crack cocaine was more addictive than powder cocaine and that individuals under its influence were more prone to crime and violence. This assertion, not based on any scientific data, but stemming from and perpetuating the vilifying and criminalizing of black and Latinx communities, was used to justify the crack versus powder cocaine sentencing disparity.

With the implementation of Reagan-era drug policies, the United States experienced the sharpest increase in its prison population in the nation's history. In 1980, approximately 300,000 individuals were incarcerated in US state and federal prisons; this number grew to more than 1.4 million by 2017.[7] As prison populations grew, racial and ethnic inequities also widened. Sixty percent of the current prison population comprises people of color, as black and Latinx people are incarcerated at disproportionately higher rates compared with their white counterparts and receive harsher sentences for similar offenses. The Fair Sentencing Act of 2010 attempted to address a major contributor to these racial disparities by eliminating the crack versus powder cocaine sentencing disparity, removing the mandatory minimum for simple cocaine possession.[8] As the bill moved through Congress, however, the Senate Judiciary Committee insisted that it only be reduced from 100:1 to 18:1, again without any scientific evidence to support harsher sentencing.[8] Although the disparate sentencing rate for crack cocaine has been reduced, this inequity remains and continues to disproportionately affect communities of color.

ADDICTION TREATMENT IN THE TWENTIETH CENTURY

Following the repeal of the National Prohibition Act in 1933, there was a period known as the "Modern Alcoholism Movement," which returned to the preprohibition concept that alcoholism was a disease and public health concern, rather than a moral failing.[9] Bill Wilson and Dr Robert Smith started Alcoholics Anonymous (AA) in 1935, with the book *Alcoholics Anonymous* being published in 1939. As AA membership grew, the organization began to expand its treatment model into private and public facilities, psychiatric hospitals, and prisons, having a major role in the return of the disease model of addiction treatment. From 1933 to 1955, the impact of the AA movement, along with the work of key professional organizations (Research Council on Problems of Alcohol, Yale Center for Alcohol Studies, and the National Committee for Education on Alcoholism), was pivotal in promoting policies that supported expanded public and private sector treatment options for individuals with alcohol addiction. Emerging out of this period, disulfiram became the first medication to receive approval from Food and Drug Administration (FDA) for treatment of addiction in 1951 (**Fig. 2**).[10]

Although treatment of unhealthy alcohol use expanded during the first half of the twentieth century, opioid addiction treatment remained largely inaccessible due to the threat of criminal penalty under the Harrison Act. This changed with the seminal 1965 study by Dole and Nyswander, which established that methadone could safely be used in the treatment of opioid addiction, providing evidence for the development of methadone maintenance therapy.[11] Legal provisions for the treatment of opioid addiction were signed into law with the Narcotic Addict Treatment Act of 1974, resulting in the establishment of Opioid Treatment Programs.[9]

The beginning of the twenty-first century signaled a shift away from harsh criminal penalties for drug possession and other drug-related offenses, toward concerted efforts to destigmatize and remedicalize the treatment of addiction. The Drug Addiction Treatment Act of 2000 waived the criminal penalty of the Harrison Narcotics Act of 1914, allowing qualified physicians to prescribe buprenorphine for the treatment of opioid use disorder in private offices and other clinical settings following its FDA approval in 2002.[9] Additional medications for the treatment of alcohol use disorder also received FDA approval, including acamprosate in 2004 and extended-release naltrexone in 2006.[10]

THE OPIOID EPIDEMIC AND RENEWED ADVOCACY EFFORTS

In the late 1990s and early 2000s, targeted marketing of opioids by the pharmaceutical industry, adoption of pain as "the fifth vital sign," minimal regulation of opioids, and a decreased appreciation of the addiction risk associated with opioid use all contributed to the second wave of the opioid epidemic (the first being heroin addiction in the late 1960s and 1970s). Opioid overdose deaths rapidly increased from 8048 in 1999 to

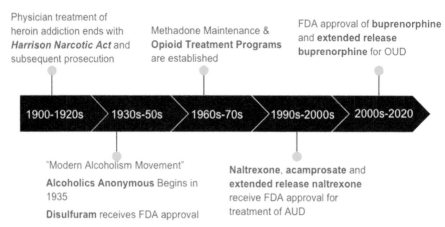

Fig. 2. Evolution of addiction treatment in the United States.

47,600 in 2017.[12] Along with deaths due to suicide and chronic liver disease, increased rates of death due to drug overdose were categorized as "deaths of despair" and cited as the major contributor to the decrease in life expectancy among middle-aged white men.[13] With a hyperfocus on increased rates of overdose deaths in white men, many other key demographics affected by this epidemic were overlooked. From 1999 to 2010, women experienced a 400% increase in rates of prescription-opioid–related deaths compared with 237% among men.[14] In addition, recent data demonstrate that rates of overdose deaths are increasing more rapidly among urban black and Latinx communities compared with whites.[15]

In the wake of this crisis, largely fueled by opioid overdose deaths in majority-white populations, media portrayals have moved away from the stereotyped, violent portrayals of addiction that plagued black communities in the 1980s and 1990s.[16] Public opinion and policies are shifting away from criminalization toward increasing access to treatment, and this change in public perception can be capitalized on to renew advocacy efforts that destigmatize, remedicalize, and decriminalize addiction.

The changing national conversation on addiction has coincided with the introduction of notable health care legislation. In 2008, Congress passed the Mental Health Parity and Addiction Equity Act, requiring insurance companies to cover mental health and addiction services equitably with respect to other health conditions.[17] Two years later, the Patient Protection and Affordable Care Act of 2010 (ACA) was passed, which allowed states to expand Medicaid eligibility for adults or children whose incomes are at or less than 138% of the federal poverty level.[18] States that expanded Medicaid through the ACA saw an increase in the number of insured individuals using addiction treatment services; however, Medicaid expansion has not demonstrated an increase in the total number of individuals enrolled in care.[19]

Despite these legislative advances, the siloing of substance use disorder care outside of traditional health care delivery systems creates barriers that result in differential access to care for some in the United States. At the time the ACA was passed, 40% of US counties did not have a substance use disorder treatment facility that accepted Medicaid.[20] Concentrated in Southern and Midwestern states, counties without a substance use disorder facility that accepted Medicaid were more likely to be rural, more likely to have higher rates of uninsured individuals, and more likely to have a higher number of black people.

DISPARITIES IN MEDICATION TREATMENT OF SUBSTANCE USE DISORDERS

Disparities in access to addiction treatment are compounded by differential rates of utilization of FDA-approved substance use disorder pharmacotherapy for some populations. Compared with privately funded substance use treatment programs, publicly funded programs are less likely to have a physician on staff and have lower rates of utilization of FDA-approved medications.[21] In addition, a nationally representative sample demonstrated that black patients were less likely than white patients to receive pharmacotherapy for alcohol use disorder.[22] Disparities in access to buprenorphine have also been demonstrated, with physician visits for opioid use disorder treatment being heavily concentrated among white and private pay patients.[23] The intensity of these disparities is even more pronounced, considering only 18% of individuals who need addiction treatment actually receive it.[2] Thus, among the 1 in 5 patients who receive treatment, those who are nonwhite or have fewer economic resources are even less likely to receive FDA-approved medications to treat addiction.

SOLUTIONS TO ADDRESS PERSISTENT DISPARITIES

As past and present drug policy and health care legislation demonstrates, policies can indeed affect various communities differently, thus creating conditions in which health inequities arise. With reinvigorated advocacy initiatives to address addiction, attention must be given to the various structural factors that shape how policy is implemented, to ensure that health care delivery systems are intentional in their advancement of health equity. The next section of this article focuses on characterizing components of equitable treatment and barriers therein, followed by recommendations and potential solutions for addressing persisting health inequities in addiction treatment.

COMPONENTS OF EQUITABLE ADDICTION TREATMENT

Addiction treatment consists of a multitude of approaches encompassing both behavioral therapies and pharmacotherapy. The National Institute of Drug Abuse details 11 principles of effective treatment, which include the acknowledgment that addiction is a complex but treatable disease and that no single treatment is appropriate for all persons.[24] Key principles relevant to addiction treatment with a health equity focus underscore that treatment (1) needs to be readily available, (2) must attend to multiple needs of the individual and not just substance use, (3) should be of adequate duration, and (4) include effective medications, in combination with culturally informed counseling and other behavioral therapies, if available.

Readily available access to treatment of substance use disorder can determine whether a patient who is prepared to address their addiction can follow through on their choice and capitalize on the often short window of motivation and action. Timely treatment early in the course of illness can potentially curb the burden of negative outcomes of a substance use disorder, including co-occurring disorder morbidity. The concept of "no wrong door" within health care systems is one approach that mitigates the access barrier. Treatment duration, often cited as a minimum of 3 months to support a reduction or cessation of substance use, should be coupled with strategic approaches to treatment reengagement, as individuals may prematurely terminate their participation in treatment services offered. Potential contributions to a lapse in treatment can be addressed through proactive assessment of services for the multiple needs of persons with substance use disorders, which often include unstable housing, food insecurity, exposures to violence, institutional racism, discrimination, and poverty, among others. These factors, often referred to as social determinants of health,[25] can drive the perpetuation of the negative outcomes from substance use disorders.

When individuals attempt to engage in treatment alongside efforts to address the social determinants, they have the highest chance of success. For people with opioid use disorders, medication for addiction treatment (MAT) should be offered first, with evidence-based therapies, when available along with comprehensive community-based supports. Services offered must adapt to the sociocultural context in which the individual resides, as treatment dropouts can result from treatment resources that fail to account for patients' diverse backgrounds and help-seeking behaviors.

BARRIERS WITHIN ADDICTION TREATMENT

A survey of participants with substance use disorders found that patients are more likely to enter addiction treatment provided in primary care settings versus specialty treatment centers.[26] These preferences may highlight the impact of stigma and discrimination on help-seeking behaviors for substance use disorder, as well as the weight of medical decision-making of primary care physicians in screening for substance use disorder and referrals to treatment. Within primary care settings, there are several barriers to appropriate screening, diagnosis, and intervention of substance use disorder. Studies of the barriers and facilitators affecting substance use screening in primary care clinics identified multilevel targets for improving access to substance use treatment. At the *individual level*, patients express concerns[27,28] over the consequences of disclosing substance use, lack of confidentiality, and a reluctance to be labeled with a substance use disorder. One study found that nearly 85% of patients were not forthcoming when asked about substance misuse.[28]

At the *provider level*, primary care physicians express[27,28] concerns over inadequate training in addiction and a limited knowledge base. Further, physicians may be missing or misdiagnosing patients who present in primary care settings with a substance use disorder related to skepticism about treatment effectiveness, discomfort discussing substance use, and lack of adequate training in medical education.[28] Provider level negative bias toward patients with substance use disorders contributes to discriminatory practices and can result in diminished empathy, less personal engagement, and the provision of suboptimal health care.[29] Stigma among primary care physicians has contributed to health disparities for patients with substance use disorders.[29] There are also *system level* concerns expressed by physicians such as time constraints, too few resources, and limited options for referrals to treatment.[27,28]

Substance use treatment has traditionally been offered by psychiatrists and allied health professionals with specialized training. However, the psychiatric workforce has a projected shortage of more than 21,000 full-time equivalent (FTE) psychiatrists by 2030.[30] As the foremost experts in the treatment of substance use disorders and co-occurring disorders, these data further demonstrate the need for innovative approaches to substance use disorder services that can extend the reach of psychiatrists into primary care settings. With increasing attention being paid to the opioid epidemic, there has been a persistent effort to improve the knowledge base of nonpsychiatrist physicians. Newly established Accreditation Council for Graduate Medical Education subspecialty programs in addiction medicine are projected to reach 125 programs by 2025, bolstering the availability of high-quality services to patients with substance use disorders seeking treatment.

As we endeavor to increase the workforce supply to meet ever-growing demands, we must also attend to the pervasive and troubling disparities in access and utilization of substance use treatment. These avoidable differences for patients with substance use disorders are stark against a backdrop of overall limited access and utilization, making the disparity an urgent matter to address. Achieving health equity for patients with substance use disorders will require targeted interventions to address several disparities: location (urban vs rural), race and ethnicity, sexual orientation, gender, language, immigration status, and age. This urgency can be addressed through new models of clinical care to tackle reduced access and engagement in care for underserved populations and others with substance use disorders.

NEW MODELS OF CLINICAL CARE

A strong evidence base supports the creation of integrated services to match the needs of patients with substance use disorders.[28] Integrating services for primary care, mental health, and substance use–related problems produces the best outcomes and provides the most effective approach for supporting whole-person health and wellness.[31] This conceptual framework for systems is essential for addressing health inequities for persons with substance use disorders. When substance-use–related services are synthesized with primary care services, they can be made available for individuals navigating addiction who are often overrepresented in general health care settings.

Targeted systematic approaches for reducing health disparities within an integrated setting include (1) having adequate resources available to screen substance use disorders, (2) capacity for delivering prevention services, (3) an ability to flexibly engage patients with substance use disorders into treatment in a timely fashion, and (4) coordination of health care services with social service systems to retain patients in treatment. Foundational policy and structural changes over the last decade in health care can support efforts for the integration of primary care and substance use services. These changes include the development of medical homes,[32] the use of information technology in accountable care organizations, and the availability of MAT in primary care settings.

Expanding access to expertise in addiction, specifically for substance use disorder subpopulations that historically navigate numerous barriers to treatment, can also be achieved through the use of psychiatric consultants. This role allows for increased reach in primary care settings through targeted screening, diagnosis, and treatment in models such as collaborative care. With a collaborative care approach, as seen in, the psychiatrist coordinates population-based services in partnership with the behavioral health manager, primary care physician, allied health professions, and behavioral health clinicians, who are all in contact with the patient. Collaborative care models have been shown to increase the proportion of patients receiving addiction treatment with remission at 6 months.[33]

Advanced Nurse Practitioners

Allied health professionals can serve as an additional front line for increased access to substance use disorder screening, diagnosis, and treatment. A recent partnership between the American Society of Addiction Medicine and the American Association of Colleges of Nursing represents a significant step toward increasing the knowledge base and skills of nurse practitioners (NPs) and is supported by grant funding from the Substance Abuse and Mental Health Services Administration. The pilot program, Nurse Practitioner Substance Use Disorder Medical Education Project, encompasses clear objectives[34] to reduce stigma around substance use disorders and increase addiction providers through the development and piloting of a curriculum designed for university NP programs on identifying and treating substance use disorders.

Culturally Sensitive Services

Culturally sensitive services, often defined as being responsive to the ethnic and cultural characteristics, experiences, norms, values, behavioral patterns, and beliefs of a target population of a treatment program,[35] are an integral aspect of many health systems, including those who provide substance use treatment. Resnicow and colleagues[35] articulate 2 dimensions of cultural sensitivity: (1) surface structure, defined as the superficial aspects of services and resources such as matching the intervention materials to the characteristics of a target population and (2) deep structure, which incorporates the cultural, historical, environmental, social, and psychological forces that influence a target health behavior within a defined population. Treatment engagement may therefore be contingent on the perceived salience of services offered, which is partially determined through deep structure assessments by patients during a consultation. A systematic review and meta-analysis of the availability of culturally sensitive youth substance use disorder services found that those with culturally sensitive treatments were associated with larger reductions in postintervention substance use rates.[36]

Given the importance of culturally informed services, federal agencies have developed resources with a directed goal of improving the quality of care delivered to specific cultural groups through cultural competence guidelines,[37] as well as treatment improvement protocols geared toward American Indian and Alaskan Natives,[38] women,[39] and sexual and gender minorities.[40] These cultural competence guidelines provide an opportunity to overcome a plethora of cultural and linguistic barriers, which have been demonstrated extensively in the literature as major deterrents to care.[41–44] Existing service structures can adopt these guidelines to improve treatment initiation and engagement among varying racial, ethnic, gender, and sexual minority groups. A sample of programs that have successfully addressed barriers to access through innovation in integrated care, use of the psychiatric consultant, allied health professionals, as well as culturally and linguistically sensitive programming has been discussed later.

EVIDENCED-BASED CARE IN ADDICTION TREATMENT

A key component of providing equitable addiction treatment is the ability to translate research approaches to clinical practice. Simply offering these treatments, without paying special attention to drug policies, historical legacies, and special cultural considerations, can often lead to dismal results. Previous research has highlighted the limited use of buprenorphine among all patients, but especially among black and Latinx patients, despite access to insurance through Medicaid.[23] Therefore, it is imperative to examine the practical implementation considerations of these interventions described later, which have largely been integrated into or interface with traditional clinical practices, given initial success in a research context. Successful implementation of all 4 models takes into consideration the institutional, personally mediated, and individual factors that can affect the utilization of addiction treatment.

The first model, known as the Vermont hub-and-spoke model,[45] was developed to address a dearth of opioid treatment providers in the state, including rural areas, where there were no addiction treaters to provide MAT. In 2000, Vermont was 1 of 8 states without opioid treatment, requiring residents to travel to neighboring states to access evidenced-based care.[45] In 2002, the first opioid treatment program (OTP) in Vermont was created, thus necessitating the recruitment and training of addiction providers, who could quickly scale up to provide medications for opioid use disorder. In this context, the hub-and-spoke model was created and successfully implemented throughout the state. Vermont was organized into 5 geographic regions, with the hub corresponding to 1 of these 5 places, that each contained an OTP. From a structural standpoint, training was enacted so that staff at each hub could accurately and safely assess a patient's medical and psychiatric needs on arrival and determine the best treatment placement.[45] The spoke associated with each hub were buprenorphine providers who had direct access to hub staff and could easily interact with other institutions, such as mental health services, emergency rooms, residential services, department of corrections, etc. The deliberate focus on the needs of the state, structural factors therein, and optimizing limited resources for the coordination of care led to a successful effort that was rapidly optimized to provide state-level addiction care in a short amount of time, with substantial improvements in the availability of MAT.

The second model describes the work of Venner and colleagues,[46] researchers dedicated to improving the use of MAT among American Indian and Alaskan Natives with opioid use disorder. This work underscores the importance of considering personally mediated and cultural factors when attempting to develop programming that provides care to a historically marginalized group at great risk for opioid overdose deaths. Highlights from this project revealed that MAT implementation among American Indian and Alaskan Natives requires some level of involvement in traditional healing, an approach that recognizes both a Western and indigenous worldview, and uses collaborative health approaches to fully address the health disparities faced in this population.[46] Taken together, this research demonstrates that integration of cultural views is paramount for successful clinical implementation of MAT to address American Indian and Alaskan Natives with opioid use disorder. This model could provide the clinical foundation for other racial and ethnic minority groups that are hesitant to initiate treatment in traditional specialty clinics.

A third model is a culturally informed approach, called Imani Breakthrough,[47] Imani meaning *faith* in Swahili. The program specifically targets black and Latinx populations with substance use disorders known to have decreased addiction treatment initiation and engagement rates, despite worsening health disparities.[1,15] This program, held in 7 black and 2 Latinx churches throughout the state of Connecticut, is geared at strengthening trust among underrepresented minority populations, while simultaneously increasing referrals to traditional settings of care for MAT. Integrated into the Imani Breakthrough framework is a targeted focus on the Citizenship Model, which established the 5 Rs—rights, roles, responsibilities, resources, and relationships—necessary to establish recovery from substances, while also addressing vulnerabilities in the social determinants of health and emphasizing how spirituality can be a central aspect of recovery.[47] Given the relationships and inherent trust with facilitators in the church setting, Imani Breakthrough has been successful in engaging hundreds of people with substance use disorders in recovery groups, promoting a safer path for referral to addiction treatment in traditional settings of care.

The final model discussed is the substance use disorder initiative developed at Massachusetts General Hospital in 2014.[48] The system-wide substance use disorder initiative outlined a major goal of achieving equity in addiction by increasing access to treatment across care settings. To achieve this goal, 4 major areas of focus were established, encompassing major structural changes including the creation of an inpatient addiction consult/liaison service, integrated addiction champion teams within primary care, creation of a postdischarge clinic for patients with substance use disorders, and the hiring of recovery coaches.[48] As a result of these systematic efforts, there have been more timely consults for patients with substance use disorders and increased addiction treatment referrals in the community, along with an overall improvement in general internists' attitudes, preparedness, and clinical practice related to people with substance use disorders.[48] These efforts have led to an initiative that is stronger and more robust than ever, serving the needs of thousands of patients in a major urban center.

In closing, it is indeed realistic and possible to achieve mental health equity within addiction. This article outlines a roadmap of essential elements to achieve this goal. A historical appreciation of the policies that have resulted in the systematic exclusion of treatment options for populations experiencing health disparities is essential. This enables an ability to make long-lasting structural change that can result in impactful system-wide advancements. Further, forging partnerships with colleagues in primary care to treat people where they are less likely to face stigma can engage populations with substance use disorders who would otherwise not access treatment. Here, collaborating with addiction experts and allied health professionals, recovery coaches, and peer facilitators is key. Finally, an integration of cultural views is also paramount, paying special attention to racial, ethnic, and sexual and gender minorities.

ACKNOWLEDGEMENTS

Ayana Jordan's work was supported by grants from the Principal Investigator's departmental funds at Yale University [D000245.CC1487.PG00035.PJ000001.A J334.FD18] and the Yale Center for Clinical Investigation CTSA under award number KL2TR001862; and from the National Center for Advancing Translational Science (NCATS), components of the National Institutes of Health (NIH), and NIH roadmap for Medical Research. Funding for this project was made possible to Myra Mathis (in part) by grant no. 5H79TI081358 from SAMHSA. The views expressed do not necessarily reflect the official policies of the Department of Health and Human Services; nor does mention of trade names, commercial practices, or organizations imply endorsement by the U.S. government.

DISCLOSURE

The authors have nothing to disclose.

REFERENCES

1. Substance Abuse and Mental Health Services Administration. Key substance use and mental health indicators in the United States: Results from the 2018 National Survey on Drug Use and Health (HHS Publication No. PEP19-5068, NSDUH Series H-54). Rockville (MD): Center for Behavioral Health Statistics and Quality, Substance Abuse and Mental Health Services Administration. Available at: https://www.samhsa.gov/data/. Accessed January 20, 2020.
2. Substance Abuse. The Nation's number one health problem. Princeton (NJ): The Robert Wood Johnson Foundation; 2013. Available at: http://www.rwjf.org/content/dam/farm/reports/reports/2001/rwjf13550. Accessed August 29, 2019.
3. Sacco LN. "Drug enforcement in the United States: history, policy and trends," congressional research service 2014. Available at: https://fas.org/sgp/crs/misc/R43749.pdf. Accessed January 20, 2020.
4. King R. The narcotics bureau and the harrison act: jailing the healers and the sick. Yale Law J 1953;62(5):736–49.
5. Baum D. Legalize it all: How to win the war on drugs. Harper Magazine 2016. Available at: https://archive.harpers.org/2016/04/pdf/HarpersMagazine-2016-04-0085915.pdf. Accessed January 20, 2020.
6. Vagins D, McCurdy J. Cracks in the system: twenty years of the unjust federal crack cocaine law 2006. Available at: https://www.aclu.org/other/cracks-system-20-years-unjust-federal-crack-cocaine-law. Accessed March 28, 2020.
7. "Trends in U.S. Corrections," the sentencing project. Available at: https://sentencingproject.org/wp-content/uploads/2016/01/Trends-in-US-Corrections.pdf. Accessed January 20, 2020.
8. "Federal crack cocaine sentencing," the sentencing project. Available at: https://www.sentencingproject.org/wp-content/uploads/2016/01/Federal-Crack-Cocaine-Sentencing.pdf. Accessed January 20, 2020.
9. Henninger A, Sung H-E. History of substance abuse treatment. In: Bruinsma G, Weisburd D, editors. Encyclopedia of criminology and criminal justice. Springer; 2014. p. 2257–69. Available at: https://link.springer.com/referenceworkentry/10.1007/978-1-4614-5690-2_278. Accessed January 20, 2020.

10. Center for Substance Abuse Treatment. Incorporating alcohol pharmacotherapies into medical practice. Treatment improvement protocol (TIP) series 49. HHS publication No. (SMA) 09-4380. Rockville (MD): Substance Abuse and Mental Health Services Administration; 2009.

11. Dole V, Nyswander M. A medical treatment for diacetylmorphine (heroin) addiction: a clinical trial with methadone hydrochloride. J Am Med Assoc 1965; 193(8):80–4.

12. Center for Disease Control and Prevention, National Center for Health Statistics. "Multiple cause of death 1999-2017," CDC WONDER online database. 2020. Available at: https://www.drugabuse.gov/related-topics/trends-statistics/overdose-death-rates. Accessed January 20, 2020.

13. Case A, Deaton A. Rising morbidity and mortality in mid-life among White non-hispanic Americans in the 21st century. Proc Natl Acad Sci U S A 2015; 112(49):15078–83. Available at: www.pnas.org/cgi/doi/10.1073/pnas. 1518393112. Accessed January 20, 2020.

14. Ait-Daoud N, Blevins D, Khanna S, et al. Women and addiction: an update. Med Clin North Am 2019;103(4):699–711. Available at: https://doi.org/10.1016/j.mcna. 2019.03.002. Accessed January 20, 2020.

15. James K, Jordan A. The opioid crisis in black communities. J Law Med Ethics 2018;46(2):404–21. Available at: https://doi.org/10.1177/1073110518782949. Accessed January 20, 2020.

16. Yankah E. When addiction has a white face. The New York Times 2016. Available at: https://www.nytimes.com/2016/02/09/opinion/when-addiction-has-a-white-face.html. Accessed January 20, 2020.

17. Centers for Medicare and Medicaid Services. The mental health parity and Addiction equity act (MHPAEA). Atlanta (GA): Centers for Disease Control and Prevention; 2019. Available at: www.cms.gov/cciio/programs-and-initiatives/other-insurance-protections/mhpaea_factsheet.html. Accessed August 29, 2019.

18. Rosenbaum S. The Patient Protection and Affordable Care Act: implications for public health policy and practice. Public Health Rep 2011;126(1):130–5.

19. Andrews CM, Pollack HA, Abraham AJ, et al. Medicaid coverage in substance use disorder treatment after the Affordable Care Act. J Subst Abuse Treat 2019;102(3):1–7. Available at: https://doi.org/10.1016/j.jsat.2019.04.002. Accessed January 20, 2020.

20. Cummings JR, Wen H, Ko M, et al. Race/ethnicity and geographic access to Medicaid substance use disorder treatment facilities in the United States. JAMA Psychiatry 2014;71(2):190–6. Accessed January 20, 2020.

21. Abraham AJ, Knudsen HK, Rieckmann T, et al. Disparities in access to physicians and medications for the treatment of substance use disorders between publicly and privately funded treatment programs in the United States. J Stud Alcohol Drugs 2013;74(2):258–65. Accessed January 20, 2020.

22. Williams EC, Gupta S, Rubinsky AD, et al. Variation in receipt of pharmacotherapy for alcohol use disorders across racial/ethnic groups: A national study in the U.S. Veterans Health Administration. Drug Alcohol Depend 2017;178:527–33. Available at: https://doi.org/10.1016/j.drugalcdep.2017.06.011. Accessed January 20, 2020.

23. Lagisetty PA, Ross R, Bohnert A, et al. Buprenorphine Treatment Divide by Race/Ethnicity and Payment. JAMA Psychiatry 2019;76(9):979–81. Available at: https://doi.org/10.1001/jamapsychiatry.2019.0876. Accessed January 20, 2020.

24. National Institute on Drug Abuse, National Institutes of Health, U.S. Department of Health and Human Services. Principles of drug addiction treatment A research-based guide. Research based guide 2018.

25. About social determinants of health. World Health Organization. 2017. Available at: http://www.who.int/social_determinants/sdh_definition/en/. Accessed January 2, 2020.

26. Barry CL, Epstein AJ, Fiellin DA, et al. Estimating demand for primary care-based treatment for substance and alcohol use disorders. Addiction 2016;111(8): 1376–84.

27. McNeely J, Kumar PC, Rieckmann T, et al. Barriers and facilitators affecting the implementation of substance use screening in primary care clinics: a qualitative study of patients, providers, and staff. Addict Sci Clin Pract 2018;13(1):8.

28. U.S. Department of Health and Human Services (HHS), Office of the Surgeon General, Facing Addiction in America. The surgeon general's report on alcohol, drugs, and health. Washington, DC: HHS; 2016.

29. vvan Boekel LC, Brouwers EP, van Weeghel J, et al. Stigma among health professionals towards patients with substance use disorders and its consequences for healthcare delivery: systematic review. Drug Alcohol Depend 2013;131(1–2): 23–35.

30. Behavioral Health Workforce Projections, 2016-2030: Psychiatrists (Adult), Child and Adolescent Psychiatrists. 2018. Available at: https://bhw.hrsa.gov/sites/default/files/bhw/nchwa/projections/psychiatrists-2018.pdf. Accessed January 2, 2020.

31. SAMHSA-HRSA Center for Integrated Health Solutions. What is integrated care?. 2016. Available at: http://www.integration.samhsa.gov/resource/what-is-integrated-care. Accessed January 2, 2020.

32. D'Aunno T, Pollack H, Chen Q, et al. Linkages between patient-centered medical homes and addiction treatment organizations: results from a national survey. Med Care 2017;55(4):379–83.

33. Watkins KE, Ober AJ, Lamp K, et al. Collaborative care for opioid and alcohol use disorders in primary care: the summit randomized clinical trial. JAMA Intern Med 2017;177(10):1480–8.

34. Nurse Practitioner Substance Use Disorder Medical Education Project (NP-SUD-MedEd). 2019. Available at: https://www.asam.org/resources/publications/magazine/read/article/2019/10/31/asam-and-aacn-partner-to-increase-critical-addiction-training-for-nurse-practitioners. Accessed January 2, 2020.

35. Resnicow K, Soler R, Braithwaite RL, et al. Cultural sensitivity in substance use prevention. J Community Psychol 2000;28(3):271–90.

36. Steinka-fry KT, Tanner-smith EE, Dakof GA, et al. Culturally sensitive substance use treatment for racial/ethnic minority youth: A meta-analytic review. J Subst Abuse Treat 2017;75:22–37.

37. Substance Abuse and Mental Health Services Administration. Improving cultural competence. treatment improvement protocol (TIP) Series No. 59. HHS Publication No. (SMA) 14-4849. Rockville (MD): Substance Abuse and Mental Health Services Administration; 2014.

38. Substance Abuse and Mental Health Services Administration. Behavioral health services for American Indians and Alaska Natives. Treatment improvement protocol (TIP) series 61. HHS publication No. (SMA) 18- 5070EXSUMM. Rockville (MD): Substance Abuse and Mental Health Services Administration; 2018.

39. Substance Abuse and Mental Health Services Administration. Substance Abuse treatment: addressing the specific needs of women. Treatment improvement

protocol (TIP) series, No. 51. HHS publication No. (SMA) 13-4426. Rockville (MD): Substance Abuse and Mental Health Services Administration; 2009.

40. Broderick EB, Clark HW, editors. A provider's introduction to substance abuse treatment for lesbian, gay, bisexual, and transgender individuals. HHS Publication; 2012 [cited 2013 Feb 27]; No. (SMA) 12–4104.

41. Yu J, Clark LP, Chandra L, et al. Reducing cultural barriers to substance abuse treatment among Asian Americans: a case study in New York City. J Subst Abuse Treat 2009;37(4):398–406.

42. Masson CL, Shopshire MS, Sen S, et al. Possible barriers to enrollment in substance abuse treatment among a diverse sample of Asian Americans and Pacific Islanders: opinions of treatment clients. J Subst Abuse Treat 2013;44(3):309–15.

43. Pagano A. Barriers to drug abuse treatment for Latino migrants: treatment providers' perspectives. J Ethn Subst Abuse 2014;13(3):273–87.

44. Bowser BP, Bilal R. Drug treatment effectiveness: African-American culture in recovery. J Psychoactive Drugs 2001;33(4):391–402.

45. Brooklyn JR, Sigmon SC. Vermont hub-and-spoke model of care for opioid use disorder: development, implementation, and impact. J Addict Med 2017; 11(4):286.

46. Venner KL, Donovan DM, Campbell AN, et al. Future directions for medication assisted treatment for opioid use disorder with American Indian/Alaska Natives. Addict Behav 2018;86:111–7.

47. Chyrell B, Jordan A. IMANI Break Through: group and wrap around support intervention [draft project components] 2018. Accessed April 5, 2019.

48. Wakeman SE, Kanter GP, Donelan K. Institutional substance use disorder intervention improves general internist preparedness, attitudes, and clinical practice. J Addict Med 2017;11(4):308–14.

Achieving Mental Health Equity: Collaborative Care

Maga E. Jackson-Triche, MD, MSHS[a],*,
Jürgen Unützer, MD, MPH, MA[b], Kenneth B. Wells, MD, MPH[c,d,e,f]

KEYWORDS

- Collaborative care • Health equity and behavioral health • Mental health
- At-risk groups

KEY POINTS

- Collaborative care is an integrated care strategy, developed for primary care, that is effective for major behavioral health conditions.
- There is evidence that collaborative care can be effective in reducing disparities and improving health equity in behavioral health.
- Collaborative care in behavioral health has been extended to improve physical health outcomes for serious mental illness in mental specialty settings.
- Collaborative care in depression has been shown to be effective in partnerships of health and social/community settings in under-resourced communities.
- Innovations in technology, task shifting, and cultural centering hold promise for further improvements in behavioral health equity.

INTRODUCTION

Health equity is the principle that holds that optimal health is a human right, and that elimination of health disparities is a society's ethical responsibility.[1,2] With regard to behavioral health conditions, there is substantial and growing evidence that systems-based integrated approaches such as collaborative care (CC) can address health disparities resulting from the lack of equal access to effective care. This

[a] UCSF Health, UCSF Weill Institute for Neurosciences, 401 Parnassus Avenue, Suite LP 342, San Francisco, CA 94143-2211, USA; [b] Department of Psychiatry and Behavioral Sciences, University of Washington, 1959 Northeast Pacific Street, Seattle, WA 98195-6560, USA; [c] Department of Psychiatry and Biobehavioral Sciences, David Geffen School of Medicine, 10920 Wilshire Boulevard, Suite 300, Los Angeles, CA 90024-6505, USA; [d] Department of Health Policy and Management, Fielding School of Public Health, Los Angeles, CA, USA; [e] Center for Health Services and Society, Semel Institute for Neuroscience and Human Behavior, Los Angeles, CA, USA; [f] California Center for Excellence in Behavioral Health, Greater Los Angeles VA Health System, Los Angeles, CA, USA
* Corresponding author.
E-mail address: Maga.Jackson-Triche@ucsf.edu

Psychiatr Clin N Am 43 (2020) 501–510
https://doi.org/10.1016/j.psc.2020.05.008
0193-953X/20/© 2020 Elsevier Inc. All rights reserved.

psych.theclinics.com

evidence is especially well documented for common conditions such as clinical depression and anxiety.

This article reviews what is known about the impact of integrated care programs on improving health equity, with special emphasis on CC, a model with robust research evidence supporting efficacy and effectiveness relative to usual care, particularly for depression, anxiety, and comorbid medical conditions such as diabetes and heart disease.[3–5] The authors used the method of rapid literature review,[6] using index searches for CC and integrated care, behavioral health, and specific conditions, examining reviews and individual articles, and also using the experience/contacts of the authors to identify key articles on major themes. Specifically, evidence is reviewed supporting the effectiveness of CC (1) to treat behavioral health conditions of at-risk populations, such as low-income populations, racial and ethnic minorities, and other populations with particular risk for poor access, such as geriatric and rural populations; (2) to reduce disparities in access, quality of care, and outcomes; and (3) to explore the promise of innovative approaches, including incorporating priorities of at-risk communities.

WHAT IS COLLABORATIVE CARE?

Integrated care programs support primary care providers in addressing behavioral health conditions commonly seen in primary care settings by colocating behavioral health clinicians and/or having behavioral health clinicians collaborate off site.[7] CC, a form of integrated care, is distinguished by the following core principles: team-based collaboration with primary care providers, behavioral health care managers, and psychiatric consultants; a population-based focus using disease registries; evidence-based treatments such as antidepressant medications and/or psychotherapy; patient-centered goal setting; measurement-based assessment; and changing treatment of nonresponse.[8–12]

In randomized controlled trials (RCTs), CC is more effective in improving quality of care and outcomes than care as usual for treating depression and anxiety,[3,4,13] including in the context of comorbid medical conditions[10,11] and substance misuse.[14]

CC has been systematically evaluated for depression in adults,[3] including seniors,[15] and adolescents with depression.[16,17] CC principles have been used to improve medical care, especially preventive services, in specialty mental health settings for individuals with severe mental illness,[18,19] although a review indicated that there are currently few data on CC for schizophrenia.[20] Because of evidence of CC effectiveness, federal and commercial insurers have developed specific billing codes for CC[21] that are becoming widely adopted[22] and some states are beginning to develop funding mechanisms to cover CC.[23]

EFFECTIVENESS OF COLLABORATIVE CARE IN REDUCING MENTAL HEALTH DISPARITIES

Partners in Care (PIC), a group-level randomized trial of CC for depression in primary care, was one of the first studies to find that implementing CC can reduce racial and ethnic disparities in health outcomes. Geographic areas were selected to ensure enrollment of significant numbers of African American and Latinx patients. Besides improvements in quality of care for depression, patients receiving CC had improved mental health–related quality of life both during the first 2 years of the study and at a 5-year follow-up.[24,25] African American and Latinx participants in intervention clinics experienced significantly greater improvements in mental health outcomes than non-Latinx white people, which was evidence of a reduction in disparities between groups.[25,26] At 10-year follow-up, minorities in the CC arm, which facilitated access to cognitive behavior therapy, had significant improvement in mental health–related outcomes compared with care as usual.[27]

The Improving Mood–Promoting Access to Collaborative Treatment (IMPACT) study,[15] another early study of CC, conducted with 1801 depressed older adults from 8 health care organizations in 5 states, showed that CC had roughly equivalent benefits for racial and ethnic minority older adults and white people.[28] Subsequent reviews of interventions to address mental health disparities have highlighted these findings for CC.[29,30] In a recent systematic review of interventions to improve initiation of mental health care for racial and ethnic minority group patients, Lee-Tauler and colleagues[30] found increased rates of initiation of treatment (medication or psychotherapy) in 4 of the 7 studies of CC compared with care as usual.

In addition, Davis and colleagues[31] evaluated a technology-based approach to CC versus care as usual for depressed veterans in primary care and found greater improvement in outcomes for racial and ethnic minorities (ie, African American, Native American, and other minority) relative to white, predominantly male veterans. Cooper and colleagues[32] compared standard CC for major depression with culturally centered CC and found similar clinical outcome improvements, with greater increases in depression treatment with standard CC, but higher patient ratings of care and case management for those receiving culturally centered CC. Lagomasino and colleagues,[33] in a randomized trial of tailored CC versus usual care for depressed Latinx people, found improved outcomes, treatment rates, and satisfaction with the CC intervention, supporting CC effectiveness in this population. Similarly, a systematic review[34] of 15 eligible studies of CC for depression in non–English-speaking populations, most which used bilingual providers, found evidence suggesting that CC tailored for non–English speakers (primarily Spanish speaking) showed greater effectiveness with reduction of health disparities for that group. There was also evidence, in some studies, that a tailored CC approach resulted in more patients receiving preferred treatments. Of note, Njeru and colleagues,[35] in a descriptive evaluation of sites implementing CC in the Depression Improvement Across Minnesota Offering a New Direction (DIAMOND) study, found lower rates of engagement in CC for individuals requiring an interpreter, which suggests language/cultural tailoring may improve implementation. In a retrospective study of engagement in CC in an academic institution, DeJesus and colleagues[36] found higher rates of dropout for nonwhite compared with white patients, suggesting the importance of engagement/outreach to improve equity. Angstman and colleagues,[37] in a retrospective chart review, reported that, under care as usual, minority primary care patients had lower rates of treatment and worse depression screener scores on the Patient Health Questionnaire, 9-item, than white patients, whereas, under CC, both groups had similar outcomes improvement.

Bao and colleagues,[38] in the Prevention of Suicide in Primary Care Elderly: Collaborative Trial (PROSPECT) study of CC for depression, focused on suicide prevention in older adults and found that, over time, CC was more effective in improving treatment rates and clinical outcomes for less well-educated compared with well-educated older adults; however, the intervention was more effective for white people than for racial and ethnic minorities. Ell and colleagues[39] conducted a randomized trial of CC for depression versus care as usual for a cohort of low-income, largely Latinx female patients with cancer in a public sector oncology clinic. The intervention significantly improved depression outcomes, physical and mental health–related quality of life, and rates of depression treatment. Sanchez and Watt[40] found that, under CC,

Spanish-speaking Latinx people had higher rates of improvement than English-speaking Latinx people and white people.

Studies focusing on Asian Americans suggest that improvements in depression outcomes can be achieved using CC. For example, Ratzliff and colleagues[41] found that CC improved depression for Asian Americans seen in general medical clinics, including culturally sensitive clinics focused on Asian Americans. Yeung and colleagues[42] found improvement in outcomes and feasibility of CC for Chinese Americans seen in psychiatric clinics. For American Indian and Alaska Native populations, Lewis and Myhra[43] found that behavioral health services provided in primary care settings can improve outcomes, particularly when tailored to the culture of Native American populations.

Thomas and colleagues[44] called for health equity intervention research that not only explicitly addresses engagement, racism/discrimination, and social determinants but also uses that framework to guide the evaluation of interventions. Examples include adaptations to treatment engagement such as those used by the WeCare study[45] for cognitive behavior therapy in low-income, minority populations, and the Dobransky-Fasiska and colleagues[46] study, which used an engagement strategy to partner with non–mental health agencies to address depression care disparities. Using this framework is also consistent with CC principles of mental health interventions that effectively engage populations.

Other CC work informed by this framework is a set of implementation efforts in Los Angeles and New Orleans using community-partnered participatory research [47] (CPPR) to both support CC implementation across community coalitions and to evaluate its impact. The Witness for Wellness project used a multisector coalition approach to depression services with community leaders as intervention partners[48] and featured innovations such as community-generated arts to enhance engagement and reduce stigma.[49]

This approach was implemented for post-Katrina mental health recovery efforts in New Orleans, with extensive use of nonlicensed community health workers and community leaders as partners in delivering interventions.[50,51] This work built on international studies such as those in Ethiopia, which incorporated pastoral women in CC, and in India, with coalitions including women's groups and lay counselors in anxiety and depression care.[52–54]

Community Partners in Care (CPIC)[55,56] was a research study that incorporated the CPPR and Health Equity Action Research Trajectory (HEART) frameworks,[44] used participatory methodology, and attempted to directly address racism/discrimination. A Cochrane Collaborative Review identified CPIC as providing rigorous evidence of the added value of coalition building for improving the health of minority communities.[57] For under-resourced communities, CPIC compared a multisector coalition approach with an expert technical assistance approach in implementing an expanded CC model for depressed African American and Latinx clients identified across health care and non–health care settings. Findings for the coalition approach included improvement in mental health outcomes over 4-year follow-up; shorter-term reductions in behavioral health hospitalizations; reductions in homelessness risk factors[55,56,58,59]; and benefits for subgroups including men, women, minority groups, and those with serious mental illness.[60]

INNOVATIVE APPLICATIONS OF COLLABORATIVE CARE THAT MAY ADDRESS EQUITY AND DISPARITIES

A recent analysis of policy to address mental health equity[61] recommended that, beyond clinical care goals, there be explicit consideration of racial and ethnic discrimination and attention to addressing specific underlying social determinants of inequity. Other investigators have emphasized that mitigating social determinants, and other underlying factors that put communities at risk for poor mental health, is an important area for development.[62] Consistent with these recommendations, Resilient Baton Rouge, a post–Hurricane Katrina flood recovery effort, incorporated CC for depression into mental health recovery intervention activities for affected communities, including racial and ethnic minorities.[63] This initiative found the expanded CC model to be feasible for implementation at scale after a disaster. A study currently being implemented in New Orleans explicitly expands CC to include services for social determinants of health, such as addressing financial issues and responding to disaster exposure. Like CPIC, programs in different service sectors are randomized to a coalition versus individual-program technical assistance approach, with randomization of individual clients to information technology (IT)/applications (apps) informational resources either with or without coping support.[64]

With regard to innovations, IT (eg, telehealth, apps) may hold promise for improving health equity by expanding the reach of CC or its key components.[65] IT has been used to deliver CC for depression, including depression with medical comorbidity,[66] posttraumatic stress disorders,[67] and depression CC in rural settings.[68] CPIC stakeholders requested an IT approach to improve access to depression services, leading to IT-based cognitive behavior therapy psychoeducation.[69]

Other innovations relevant to health equity include expanding the health care workforce, such as adapting CC to include coaching by pharmacists,[70] and adding nurse outreach activities.[71] There is ongoing research examining applications of CC to other mental health conditions such as bipolar disorder,[68] serious mental illness,[19] and addiction.[72,73] Such studies may hold promise for expanding applications of CC to behavioral health, and for exploring its potential to reduce disparities related to these conditions.

SUMMARY

The literature cited earlier gives strong evidence for CC as a model with the potential to reduce disparities for ethnic minority and other at-risk populations who are often poorly served by usual primary care systems, and who have worse engagement and outcomes because of other underlying risk factors. As a systems-based approach, CC has been shown to not only improve access to care but also to improve the quality of care received and health outcomes.

A limitation is that the authors followed a rapid rather than systematic review process and did not attempt to identify all CC studies in behavioral health, but rather key articles in main areas that noted diverse populations or that directly addressed disparities/health equity.

The findings presented here reinforce the view that reaching mental health equity is an achievable goal and that CC can play an important role. To more fully realize the promise of CC, there is the need for approaches that focus on effective community engagement, coalition building, and cultural adaptation, as well as developing innovative approaches such as addressing social determinants. Key first steps are using health equity–focused strategies when planning and implementing CC and giving careful thought and attention to engaging diverse populations and considering their specific preferences and needs.

DISCLOSURE

The authors have nothing to disclose.

REFERENCES

1. Sanchez K, Ybarra R, Chapa T, et al. Eliminating behavioral health disparities and improving outcomes for racial and ethnic minority populations. Psychiatr Serv 2015;67(1):13–5.
2. Braveman P, Arkin E, Orleans T, et al. What is health equity? and what difference does a definition make? Princeton (NJ): Robert Wood Johnson Foundation; 2017.
3. Gilbody S, Whitty P, Grimshaw J, et al. Educational and organizational interventions to improve the management of depression in primary care: a systematic review. JAMA 2003;289(23):3145–51.
4. Gilbody S, Bower P, Fletcher J, et al. Collaborative care for depression: a cumulative meta-analysis and review of longer-term outcomes. Arch Intern Med 2006;166(21):2314–21.
5. Huffman JC, Mastromauro CA, Beach SR, et al. Collaborative care for depression and anxiety disorders in patients with recent cardiac events: the Management of Sadness and Anxiety in Cardiology (MOSAIC) randomized clinical trial. JAMA Intern Med 2014;174(6):927–35.
6. Ganann R, Ciliska D, Thomas H. Expediting systematic reviews: methods and implications of rapid reviews. Implement Sci 2010;5(1):56.
7. Ramanuj P, Ferenchik E, Docherty M, et al. Evolving Models of Integrated Behavioral Health and Primary Care. Curr Psychiatry Rep 2019;21(1):4.
8. Unützer J, Harbin H, Schoenbaum M, et al. The collaborative care model: an approach for integrating physical and mental health care in Medicaid health homes. Services CfMaM; 2013. p. 1–13.
9. Katon W, Von Korff M, Lin E, et al. Collaborative management to achieve treatment guidelines: impact on depression in primary care. JAMA 1995;273(13):1026–31.
10. Katon WJ, Von Korff M, Lin EH, et al. The Pathways Study: a randomized trial of collaborative care in patients with diabetes and depression. Arch Gen Psychiatry 2004;61(10):1042–9.
11. Katon WJ, Lin EH, Von Korff M, et al. Collaborative care for patients with depression and chronic illnesses. N Engl J Med 2010;363(27):2611–20.
12. AIMS Center. Advancing Integrated Mental Health Solutions. Available at: http://aims.uw.edu/. Accessed December 16, 2019.
13. Luxama C, Dreyfus D. Collaborative care for depression and anxiety. Am Fam Physician 2014;89(7):524–5.
14. Watkins KE, Paddock SM, Zhang L, et al. Improving care for depression in patients with comorbid substance misuse. Am J Psychiatry 2006;163(1):125–32.
15. Unützer J, Katon W, Callahan CM, et al. Collaborative care management of late-life depression in the primary care setting: a randomized controlled trial. JAMA 2002;288(22):2836–45.
16. Asarnow JR, Jaycox LH, Duan N, et al. Effectiveness of a quality improvement intervention for adolescent depression in primary care clinics: a randomized controlled trial. JAMA 2005;293(3):311–9.
17. Richardson LP, Ludman E, McCauley E, et al. Collaborative care for adolescents with depression in primary care: a randomized clinical trial. JAMA 2014;312(8):809–16.
18. Druss BG, Bradford WD, Rosenheck RA, et al. Quality of medical care and excess mortality in older patients with mental disorders. Arch Gen Psychiatry 2001;58(6):565–72.

19. Young AS, Cohen AN, Chang ET, et al. A clustered controlled trial of the implementation and effectiveness of a medical home to improve health care of people with serious mental illness: study protocol. BMC Health Serv Res 2018;18(1):428.

20. Reilly S, Planner C, Gask L, et al. Collaborative care approaches for people with severe mental illness. Cochrane Database Syst Rev 2013;(11):CD009531.

21. Press MJ, Howe R, Schoenbaum M, et al. Medicare payment for behavioral health integration. N Engl J Med 2017;376(5):405–7.

22. Carlo AD, Unützer J, Ratzliff AD, et al. Financing for collaborative care—a narrative review. Curr Treat Options Psychiatry 2018;5(3):334–44.

23. Getting Paid in the Collaborative Care Model. American Psychiatric Association. Available at: https://www.psychiatry.org/psychiatrists/practice/professional-interests/integrated-care/learn. Accessed December 16, 2019.

24. Sherbourne CD, Wells KB, Duan N, et al. Long-term effectiveness of disseminating quality improvement for depression in primary care. Arch Gen Psychiatry 2001;58(7):696–703.

25. Wells K, Sherbourne C, Schoenbaum M, et al. Five-year impact of quality improvement for depression: results of a group-level randomized controlled trial. Arch Gen Psychiatry 2004;61(4):378–86.

26. Miranda J, Duan N, Sherbourne C, et al. Improving care for minorities: can quality improvement interventions improve care and outcomes for depressed minorities? Results of a randomized, controlled trial. Health Serv Res 2003;38(2):613–30.

27. Sherbourne CD, Edelen MO, Zhou A, et al. How a therapy-based quality improvement intervention for depression affected life events and psychological well-being over time: a 9-year longitudinal analysis. Med Care 2008;46(1):78–84.

28. Areán PA, Ayalon L, Hunkeler E, et al. Improving depression care for older, minority patients in primary care. Med Care 2005;43:381–90.

29. McGuire TG, Miranda J. New evidence regarding racial and ethnic disparities in mental health: policy implications. Health Aff (Millwood) 2008;27(2):393–403.

30. Lee-Tauler SY, Eun J, Corbett D, et al. A systematic review of interventions to improve initiation of mental health care among racial-ethnic minority groups. Psychiatr Serv 2018;69(6):628–47.

31. Davis TD, Deen T, Bryant-Bedell K, et al. Does minority racial-ethnic status moderate outcomes of collaborative care for depression? Psychiatr Serv 2011;62(11):1282–8.

32. Cooper LA, Ghods Dinoso BK, Ford DE, et al. Comparative effectiveness of standard versus patient-centered collaborative care interventions for depression among African Americans in primary care settings: the BRIDGE study. Health Serv Res 2013;48(1):150–74.

33. Lagomasino IT, Dwight-Johnson M, Green JM, et al. Effectiveness of collaborative care for depression in public-sector primary care clinics serving latinos. Psychiatr Serv 2016;68(4):353–9.

34. Garcia ME, Ochoa-Frongia L, Moise N, et al. Collaborative care for depression among patients with limited english proficiency: a systematic review. J Gen Intern Med 2018;33(3):347–57.

35. Njeru JW, DeJesus RS, Sauver JS, et al. Utilization of a mental health collaborative care model among patients who require interpreter services. Int J Ment Health Syst 2016;10(1):15.

36. DeJesus R, Njeru J, Angstman K. Engagement among minority patients in collaborative care management for depression. Chron Dis Int 2015;2(1).

37. Angstman KB, Phelan S, Myszkowski MR, et al. Minority primary care patients with depression: outcome disparities improve with collaborative care management. Med Care 2015;53(1):32–7.
38. Bao Y, Alexopoulos GS, Casalino LP, et al. Collaborative depression care management and disparities in depression treatment and outcomes. Arch Gen Psychiatry 2011;68(6):627–36.
39. Ell K, Xie B, Quon B, et al. Randomized controlled trial of collaborative care management of depression among low-income patients with cancer. J Clin Oncol 2008;26(27):4488.
40. Sanchez K, Watt TT. Collaborative care for the treatment of depression in primary care with a low-income, Spanish-speaking population: outcomes from a community-based program evaluation. Prim Care Companion CNS Disord 2012;14(6). PCC.12m01385.
41. Ratzliff AD, Ni K, Chan Y-F, et al. A collaborative care approach to depression treatment for Asian Americans. Psychiatr Serv 2013;64(5):487–90.
42. Yeung A, Shyu I, Fisher L, et al. Culturally sensitive collaborative treatment for depressed Chinese Americans in primary care. Am J Public Health 2010; 100(12):2397–402.
43. Lewis ME, Myhra LL. Integrated care with indigenous populations: a systematic review of the literature. Am Indian Alsk Native Ment Health Res 2017;24(3): 88–110.
44. Thomas SB, Quinn SC, Butler J, et al. Toward a fourth generation of disparities research to achieve health equity. Annu Rev Public Health 2011;32:399–416.
45. Miranda J, Green BL, Krupnick JL, et al. One-year outcomes of a randomized clinical trial treating depression in low-income minority women. J Consult Clin Psychol 2006;74(1):99.
46. Dobransky-Fasiska D, Nowalk MP, Pincus HA, et al. Public-academic partnerships: improving depression care for disadvantaged adults by partnering with non-mental health agencies. Psychiatr Serv 2010;61(2):110–2.
47. Jones L, Wells K. Strategies for academic and clinician engagement in community-participatory partnered research. JAMA 2007;297(4):407–10.
48. Bluthenthal RN, Jones L, Fackler-Lowrie N, et al. Witness for Wellness: preliminary findings from a community-academic participatory research mental health initiative. Ethn Dis 2006;16(1):S1.
49. Chung B, Jones L, Jones A, et al. Using community arts events to enhance collective efficacy and community engagement to address depression in an African American Community. Am J Public Health 2009;99(2):237–44.
50. Springgate BF, Wennerstrom A, Meyers D, et al. Building community resilience through mental health infrastructure and training in post-Katrina New Orleans. Ethn Dis 2011;21(3 0 1):S1.
51. Wennerstrom A, Vannoy SD, Allen CE, et al. Community-based participatory development of a community health worker mental health outreach role to extend collaborative care in post-Katrina New Orleans. Ethn Dis 2011;21(3 0 1):S1.
52. Coppock DL, Desta S, Tezera S, et al. Capacity building helps pastoral women transform impoverished communities in Ethiopia. Science 2011;334(6061): 1394–8.
53. Tripathy P, Nair N, Barnett S, et al. Effect of a participatory intervention with women's groups on birth outcomes and maternal depression in Jharkhand and Orissa, India: a cluster-randomised controlled trial. Lancet 2010;375(9721): 1182–92.

54. Patel V, Weiss HA, Chowdhary N, et al. Effectiveness of an intervention led by lay health counsellors for depressive and anxiety disorders in primary care in Goa, India (MANAS): a cluster randomised controlled trial. Lancet 2010;376(9758): 2086–95.

55. Wells KB, Jones L, Chung B, et al. Community-partnered cluster-randomized comparative effectiveness trial of community engagement and planning or resources for services to address depression disparities. J Gen Intern Med 2013; 28(10):1268–78.

56. Chung B, Ong M, Ettner SL, et al. 12-month cost outcomes of community engagement versus technical assistance for depression quality improvement: a partnered, cluster randomized, comparative-effectiveness trial. Ethn Dis 2018; 28(Suppl 2):349–56.

57. Anderson LM, Adeney KL, Shinn C, et al. Community coalition-driven interventions to reduce health disparities among racial and ethnic minority populations. Cochrane Database Syst Rev 2015;(6):CD009905.

58. Chung B, Ngo VK, Ong MK, et al. Participation in training for depression care quality improvement: a randomized trial of community engagement or technical support. Psychiatr Serv 2015;66(8):831–9.

59. Arevian AC, Jones F, Tang L, et al. Depression remission from community coalitions versus individual program support for services: findings from community partners in Care, Los Angeles, California, 2010-2016. Am J Public Health 2019; 109(S3):S205–13.

60. Castillo EG, Shaner R, Tang L, et al. Improving depression care for adults with serious mental illness in underresourced areas: community coalitions versus technical support. Psychiatr Serv 2018;69(2):195–203.

61. Miranda J, Snowden LR, Legha RK. Policy Effects on Mental Health Status and Mental Health Care Disparities. In: Goldman HH, Frank RG, Morrissey JP, editors. The palgrave handbook of American mental health policy. Cham (Switzerland): Palgrave Macmillan; 2020. p. 331–66.

62. Hoeft TJ, Wilcox H, Hinton L, et al. Costs of implementing and sustaining enhanced collaborative care programs involving community partners. Implement Sci 2019;14(1):37.

63. Keegan R, Grover L, Patron D, et al. Case study of resilient baton rouge: applying depression collaborative care and community planning to disaster recovery. Int J Environ Res Public Health 2018;15(6):1208.

64. Springgate B, Arevian A, Wennerstrom A, et al. Community resilience learning collaborative and research network (C-LEARN): study protocol with participatory planning for a randomized, comparative effectiveness trial. Int J Environ Res Public Health 2018;15(8):1683.

65. Pyne JM, Fortney JC, Tripathi SP, et al. Cost-effectiveness analysis of a rural telemedicine collaborative care intervention for depression. Arch Gen Psychiatry 2010;67(8):812–21.

66. Rollman BL, Belnap BH, LeMenager MS, et al. Telephone-delivered collaborative care for treating post-CABG depression: a randomized controlled trial. JAMA 2009;302(19):2095–103.

67. Fortney JC, Pyne JM, Mouden SB, et al. Practice-based versus telemedicine-based collaborative care for depression in rural federally qualified health centers: a pragmatic randomized comparative effectiveness trial. Am J Psychiatry 2013; 170(4):414–25.

68. Fortney JC, Pyne JM, Kimbrell TA, et al. Telemedicine-based collaborative care for posttraumatic stress disorder: a randomized clinical trial. JAMA Psychiatry 2015;72(1):58–67.

69. Arevian AC, O'Hora J, Jones F, et al. Participatory technology development to enhance community resilience. Ethn Dis 2018;28(Suppl 2):493–502.

70. Brook O, van Hout H, Nieuwenhuyse H, et al. Impact of coaching by community pharmacists on drug attitude of depressive primary care patients and acceptability to patients; a randomized controlled trial. Eur Neuropsychopharmacol 2003;13(1):1–9.

71. Dick J, Clarke M, Van Zyl H, et al. Primary health care nurses implement and evaluate a community outreach approach to health care in the South African agricultural sector. Int Nurs Rev 2007;54(4):383–90.

72. Watkins KE, Ober AJ, Lamp K, et al. Collaborative care for opioid and alcohol use disorders in primary care: the SUMMIT randomized clinical trial. JAMA Intern Med 2017;177(10):1480–8.

73. Saitz R, Cheng DM, Winter M, et al. Chronic care management for dependence on alcohol and other drugs: the AHEAD randomized trial. JAMA 2013;310(11):1156–67.

Achieving Mental Health Equity: Community Psychiatry

Jacqueline Maus Feldman, MD*

KEYWORDS

- Community mental health • Stigma reduction • Disparities • Mental health equity

KEY POINTS

- Community mental health inequities exist and are predicated on stigma related to mental illness.
- Inequities exist in funding of training, research, and service.
- Inequities lead to deficits in workforce development, access to care, and increased morbidity and mortality.
- To remedy these deficits, there must be adequate funding; appropriate training of adequate numbers of recovery-oriented, culturally competent, and trauma-informed providers; and use of consistent evidence-based care.

INTRODUCTION

In 2003, the Institute of Medicine, commenting on "Unequal Treatment," defined "disparity" as a "difference in healthcare quality not due to differences in health care needs or preferences of the patient." In the United States, the provision and receipt of community mental health care is replete with disparities. These disparities are predicated on an abysmal history of stigma and discrimination, which has resulted in the philosophic embrace and practice of unequal care for those living with mental illness. There are disparities within disparities of unequal access and care for people of different ethnicities. Dire consequences have followed for individuals, families, facilities, systems of care, and communities, including excessive morbidity and mortality; overwhelmed outpatient clinics, emergency rooms, and hospitals; and the use of the criminal justice system in lieu of support and treatment.[1]

Despite these challenges, solutions and models of care exist that may facilitate mental health equity within the community. Stigma reduction, legislative/judicial

Department of Psychiatry and Behavioral Neurobiology, University of Alabama at Birmingham, Birmingham, AL, USA
* SC 560, 1720 2nd Avenue, Birmingham, AL 35294-0017.
E-mail address: Jfeldman@uabmc.edu

Psychiatr Clin N Am 43 (2020) 511–524
https://doi.org/10.1016/j.psc.2020.06.002
0193-953X/20/© 2020 Elsevier Inc. All rights reserved.

psych.theclinics.com

Abbreviations
ACE   adverse childhood experiences
APA   American Psychiatric Association

---

intervention, workforce development, improved access, prevention, early identification, attention to social determinants, and adequate funding could go a long way in mitigating the effects of mental health disparities in the community.

HISTORICAL PERSPECTIVES IN COMMUNITY MENTAL HEALTH DISPARITIES

Since the founding of the United States, those living with mental illness have been subject to prejudice, stigma, and discrimination. In early America, consideration of those with mental illness focused on the perception of their being possessed by demons, prone to evil spirits, and having a predilection for violence. "Treatment" consisted of isolation, restraint, sedation, and ultimately institutionalization. Before the mid 1800s, these folks were hidden in attics or basements, or cast out to fend for themselves, and many families and most organized leadership entities (churches and local, state, and federal governments) rejected responsibility for their care. Although those with communicable diseases were treated with whatever limited medical means were available, those with mental illness were judged as undeserving of health care. Mental illness was considered discrete from medical illness, justifying mistreatment, or found to be undeserving of any treatment at all.[2]

In America, the mid 1800s brought forward the European concept of "moral treatment," advocated for by Dorthea Dix, who spent years lobbying first the federal government (President Franklin Pierce in 1854 ultimately refused to accept federal responsibility for the provision of mental health care), then individual state governments to create institutions that would provide milieus of support and treatment; moral treatment entailed provision of safe and nurturing environments, peaceful surroundings, nutritious diets, and productive work in institutions found in placid rural settings. Unfortunately, these establishments were soon inundated by other less fortunate in society (victims of infectious disease, wayward wives, the impoverished, abandoned children), such that state hospital populations reached more than 550,000 by 1950; state hospital care devolved in many locations to custodial care at best, with limited funding, staff, and treatment options, including hydrotherapy, electroconvulsive therapy, and insulin shock. A focus on psychoanalysis proved helpful to limited numbers of patients (and was not accessible to the general population). Some advancements in diagnosis (increasing observance of stress-related wartime changes in behavior) barely nudged public understanding of mental health. The arena of mental illness continued to receive limited attention, funding, research, and those living with mental illness had, at best, few treatment options; at worst, they were ignored, neglected, and abandoned. In the late 1940s and 1950s, some hope was generated by the National Mental Health Act of 1948, which led to the creation of the National Institutes of Mental Health, and the discovery of medication (antipsychotics and mood stabilizers) that could impact mental illness. The Mental Retardation Facilities and Community Mental Health Center Construction Act was signed into law in 1963, and was to begin the grand process of planning and funding an extensive community outpatient care network. The initiation of Medicaid and Medicare was potentially a turning point for mental health care. Unfortunately, a flood of deinstitutionalizations from state hospitals with insufficient funding for local inpatient or outpatient care, an inadequate workforce, and ongoing stigma resulted in the perpetuation of mental health care disparities. The 1980s opened the door to improvement in pharmaceutical treatment (clozapine, atypical antipsychotics, new generations of mood stabilizers), but limited state and federal funding of treatment centers continued to plague access to care. The separation of substance use disorders from other mental illness also complicated access and treatment. Present throughout was ongoing societal stigma related to mental illness, and perpetually constrained budgets, which contributed to ongoing arguments over who was responsible for care. Disparities in funding for workforce development, and access to adequate and appropriate treatment continued to plague systems of care, and the individuals they were meant to serve.[3]

MODERN-DAY INEQUITIES

To better understand the consequences of present-day health disparities, a review of national statistics that reflect the current realities of limited workforce, the stark and massive unmet mental health needs, and inadequate services is in order.

The boxes in this article identify the challenges people living with mental illness face. **Box 1** frames the population needs using demographics and statistics.

Box 1
Framing the population needs

One in 5 Americans will experience mental illness in a given year.[11,23]

One-half of all Americans are living with a diagnosable mental illness at some point during their life.[11]

Twenty percent of children currently or at some point in their life have had a seriously debilitating mental disorder.[24]

One in 25 Americans live with a serious mental illness (such as schizophrenia, bipolar disorder, or major depression).[23]

One in 10 women experience depression sometime during their life, 1 in 9 of those who have been pregnant have symptoms of postpartum depression.[24]

Mental illnesses, such as depression, are the third most common cause of hospitalization in the United States for those aged 18 to 44.[24]

Those with poor mental health have an increased risk of heart disease, stroke, and cancer; 17% of adults have comorbid physical and behavioral health issues.[23,24]

Those living with schizophrenia are at risk of dying 25 years earlier than the general population.[24]

More than one-half of American adults with diagnosable mental illness do not receive mental health care.[25]

The average delay between the onset of mental illness symptoms and treatment is 11 years.[23]

Only 33% of Latinos and 31% of African Americans receive the requisite mental health or substance use care.[23]

More than 50% of patients receive their behavioral health treatment from primary care sources, who may not have adequate behavioral health care training.[26,27]

People with behavioral health issues have 2 to 3 times the health care costs of those who do not. It has been suggested that for every $1 expended on behavioral health savings of $4 to 5 dollars could occur on the medical side.[18]

Per the World Economic Forum, mental disorders are the largest cost driver in global costs in 2010 ($2.5 trillion); projected to be 16 trillion by 2030.[28]

Data from Refs.[11,18,23–28]

Considerable numbers of Americans live with mental illness, and are vulnerable to serious complications, but are unable to access quality care within an adequate timeframe.

The **Boxes 2–4** denote deficits in the numbers of skilled mental health providers, adequate funding, and appropriate services. There are an increasingly limited number of mental health providers willing and able to see community outpatient mental health populations, and there are inadequate mechanisms to build a competent workforce. If one lives in a rural area and needs mental health services, there may be no available providers; if one lives in an urban area, one will most likely experience long wait lists. Access to hospital beds is plummeting, and many emergency rooms are unable to respond appropriately to patients requiring mental health services.

Consequences of Modern-Day Inequities

The state of community mental health care in 2020 continues to reflect the challenges of mental health disorders[4]; stigma and discrimination for those living with mental illness remain rampant and manifest in many ways. Local, state, and federal funding for mental health treatment is haphazard, resulting in limited research, incomplete workforce (in numbers and competencies), inadequate prevention, missed opportunities for early identification, insufficient and unresponsive access, limited supports,

---

Box 2
Dwindling numbers of psychiatric providers

From 1995 to 2013, the number of adult psychiatrists and child and adolescent psychiatrists increased by only 12%, compared with the 45% increase in total physician numbers and population growth.[29]

There are 28,250 psychiatrists are in active practice in the United States, but they are unevenly distributed; most are in California, New York, Texas, Pennsylvania, and Florida.[30]

By 2020, there will be 12,624 child and adolescent psychiatrists needed, far exceeding the anticipated supply of more than 8300.[31]

Currently, 59% of psychiatrists are 55 years of age or older (raising the harbinger of upcoming retirements without replacement providers).[29]

There are 89.3 million Americans who live in federally designated Mental Health Professional Shortage Areas (compared with 55.3 million living in primary care shortage areas). There is a shortage of 2800 psychiatrists in rural and underserved areas. It is believed with the increasing geriatric population, that without workforce development, there will be only 1 geriatric psychiatrist for every 6000 geriatric patients living with mental illness or substance use disorder.[4]

Seventy-seven percent of US counties report severe deficiencies in psychiatrists.[32]

The number of psychiatry residency training positions has been slowly increasing since 2013; in 2019 there were 1740 slots available (this represents 4.9% of total residency slots); 1720 slots were awarded.[33]

The shortage of psychiatrists has been exacerbated by the Federal Funding Balanced Budget Act of 1997, which placed caps on federal funding of residency programs.[34]

Although reflecting 13% and 14%, respectively, of the general American population, only 3% of active psychiatrists are African American and 2% of psychologists; 5% of psychiatrists are Latino and 3% of psychologists are Latino. All told, only 21% of psychiatric care comes from providers with diverse backgrounds.[35]

Data from Refs.[4,29–35]

Box 3
Decreases in funding for psychiatric services

Salaries in behavioral health professions are well below comparable positions in other health care sectors. The median compensation for psychiatry is the third lowest among 30 medical specialties. Reimbursements (private insurance, federal payors) do not cover provider costs.[31]

Low wages and benefits, heavy caseloads, and stigma associated with working with these populations are cited as disincentives to being engaged in community mental health. Psychiatrists report underpayment by private insurance, and paperwork required by Medicare as motivators to change the source of their revenue stream.[36]

From 2005 to 2010, the percentage of psychiatrists who accepted private insurance decreased by 17% points to 55%. The percentage of psychiatrists accepting Medicare decreased by 20% points to 55%. Unfortunately, by running cash-only based practices, they limit the numbers (and kinds) of patients they are willing to treat.[37]

Whites are the only racial group in which the majority of people with severe psychiatric distress get treatment. Overall spending for African Americans and Latinos on outpatient mental health care is 60% to 75% of spending for whites.[38,39]

All minority groups are less likely to be covered by health insurance. They will have less capacity to access mental health services, are less likely to receive care, and are more likely to receive poor quality care.[40,41]

Medicaid is the single largest source of funding for behavioral health care in the country. Not every state has expanded Medicaid.[31]

Data from Refs.[31,36–41]

early mortality, and transinstitutionalization. The capacity for developing resilience in the face of early childhood adverse experiences, traumatic stress (including military and disaster responses), and adverse climate change also impact on vulnerable communities.

Box 4
Paucity of services

Only 27% of the nation's community hospitals contain a separate inpatient psychiatric unit, down 80% from 40 years ago.[42,43]

Seventy percent of 6000 surveyed emergency rooms reported boarding psychiatric patients who were waiting for an inpatient bed for prolonged time periods (>24 hours).[4,44]

Sixty-one percent of emergency rooms do not have psychiatric staff caring for patients in the emergency room while boarding.[4]

In 1955, nationwide there were 340 public psychiatry beds (state hospital beds) per 100,000 general population; by 2005 it had decrease by 95% to 17 per 100,000. The authors suggested a minimal acceptable number is closer to 50 per 100,000. Of the 50 states, 42 had less than one-half the minimum suggested.[43]

Racial and ethnic minorities are less likely to get the preventative care they need to stay healthy, are more likely to suffer from serious illness, and when sick are less likely to have access to quality health care.[45]

The Surgeon General report in 1999 noted that racial and ethnic minorities have less access to mental health services, are less likely to receive medical care, and are more likely to receive poor quality care. They are more likely to delay or fail to seek care, and are more likely to terminate care.[7]

Data from Refs.[4,7,42–45]

Stigma

People living with mental illness face considerable barriers because of stigma. Stigma results from the negative reaction of the public to those living with mental illness. The predicates to stigma include stereotyping ("negative beliefs held about a group"), and prejudice ("agreement with a belief and/or a negative emotional reaction"), which often lead to discrimination.[5] Research reflects that stigma in the Western world related to mental illness is often sanctioned by the general public, and that discrimination can promulgate behaviors that include avoidance (because of fear), authoritarianism (those with mental illness are irresponsible and should have life decisions made for them), or benevolence (those with mental illness are like children and need protection). Ultimately, this can be translated into withholding help, coercing treatment, or insisting on segregation. For example, such stigma might trigger an emergency room's refusal to treat patients living with serious mental illness, instead referring them into the criminal justice system. It might rob them "of the opportunities that define a quality life: good jobs, safe housing, satisfactory health care, and affiliation with a diverse group of people."[5]

Funding

Funding for the provision of mental health services has not kept pace with funding for the provision of physical medical care. The passage of the Mental Health Parity and Addiction Equity Act of 2008 was designed to impose standards of equitable payment for mental health services (eg, doctors providing Medicare-funded services could not charge different copays; previously, Medicare mental health patients were having to pay 50% copays vs 20% copays for medical services), and life-time maximums could not be different. However, it took several years to get final regulations in place, and ongoing court cases still reflect the nation's insurance companies are resistant to equity in funding care. The Affordable Care Act of 2010 mandated that insurance must cover mental health care (in the past insurance had embraced an "exceptionalism" philosophy, reflecting their fears that mental health service costs would become excessive, hence payment for services was limited (caps on numbers of outpatient visit, inpatient days, higher copays). More recent research reflects that an integrated approach (equivalence of payments for medical and psychiatric care) has not resulted in excessive mental health costs. In the National Survey on Drug Use and Health (2008–2012) by the Substance Abuse and Mental Health Services Administration, cost was the most commonly cited reason for why individuals of any ethnicity chose to not use mental health or substance abuse services.[6]

Research

US data from 2011 reflect that the top 3 deadliest (most deaths) diseases were heart disease, chronic obstructive pulmonary disease, and diabetes mellitus; however, they respectively received only the third, sixth, and seventh levels of research funding.[7] Breast and prostate cancer, responsible for many fewer deaths, were first and second in funding. Although suicide was the cause of an estimated 40,000 deaths, it was the least funded disease entity, receiving 100 times less than breast cancer.[8] This has improved over the years; by 2019, National Institutes of Health funding for breast cancer research was US$709 million, whereas suicide US$177 million. Across the spectrum of mental illness, inequalities remain: one might notice a discordance between the numbers of people affected or cost burden of disease and research dollars spent as one reviews the 2019 National Institutes of Health research funding (in millions of dollars): Alzheimer's (2,240), opioids (978), depression (578), schizophrenia (263), anxiety (233), and post-traumatic stress disorder (138).[9]

Prevention

Mental Health America issued a report in 2019[10] on prevention and early intervention, noting that one-half of those who become affected by mental illness develop symptoms by age 14. Without active intervention, significant consequences can occur. Adverse childhood experiences (ACEs) such as abuse, neglect, sexual trauma, violence, and/or exposure to violence can play a pivotal role in the development of mental health issues. Interruptions in access to housing, food, education, and physical or mental health care can prove incredibly troublesome to these vulnerable populations. Relationship disruptions (isolation, bullying) often impact on children and adolescents. Failure to identify and intercede when children are confronted with the aforementioned challenges can have serious consequences including:

- Suicide (a study of ninth to twelfth grades reflected an 8% report of suicide attempts during the prior year)
- Incarceration (there are 600,000 youth engaged in the juvenile justice system, 65%–70% with a diagnosable mental illness; 90% have been exposed to ACEs, many of them to ≥ 6 ACEs).
- Homelessness
- School dropouts (1 in 10 of those who drop out before graduating ends up spending some time institutionalized; by comparison, 1 in 13 of high school graduates, and 1 in 500 who receive college degrees share the same fate).[10]

Early Identification

Multiple studies have underscored the importance of early identification and then treatment.[11,12] In particular, the literature is replete with the effectiveness of accessing early intervention in psychosis. National funding has supported the development of early intervention teams that provide not only assessments, but also long-term treatment plans that include medication, individual and family therapy, cognitive remediation, education, and vocational support. Without early identification (which means parents, educators, and health providers act as sentinels), illness can proceed unabated and make later attempts at treatment more challenging.

Limited Access

As noted in **Boxes 1–4**, there are often multiple barriers to accessing mental health care. In addition to stigma and insufficient funding, limited numbers of health care providers, or providers who lack cultural competencies or clinical expertise, can limit the impact of care. Waiting for an outpatient appointment (which can take days, weeks, and even months) is frustrating, and can be dangerous in terms of suicide or disease progression. Emergency rooms are often considered the only access into a system of care, but can lead to prolonged boarding times and placement in distant hospitals. Discharges from psychiatric inpatient units are often complicated by the lack of accessible outpatient care. Without access to care, clinical presentations may worsen; often, untreated patients can become so ill they act out in an aggressive or psychotic fashion, and the criminal justice system becomes the route to "treatment" (incarceration where psychiatric care may be extremely limited)

Limited Supports

Limited resources in one's life can negatively impact a person/family in many ways. Unemployment means limited income, and hence a limited capacity to pay for housing, nutrition, and health care, including prescriptions. Limited transportation can complicate accessing appointments, which in turn can lead to nonadherence with treatment.

Workforce

As noted in **Boxes 2** and **3**, there are significant holes in the workforce necessary to offer community mental health care. There simply are not enough psychiatrists to care for the numbers of people living with mental illness, and long wait times are common. It was reported that by decreasing the wait times in outpatient mental health practices from 13 to 0 days, no show rates decreased from 52% to 18%.[13] An inadequately trained workforce (in terms of cultural competence) providing services in clinics that do not reflect the treatment population's values or language can negatively impact opportunities for engagement and appropriate treatment.[14]

Morbidity and Mortality

With insufficient care, psychiatric patients may decompensate further, or relapse. This can lead to further complications (eg, suicide, violence, aggression, arrest and incarceration, substance use, job loss, and relationship disruptions).

Transinstitutionalization

Hundreds of thousands of patients have been released from state hospitals since the mid 1960s. With insufficient supports in place (ie, housing, outpatient clinics, adequate income) people living with mental illness became homeless, were placed in nursing homes, or became incarcerated. There are more people living with serious mental illness being served in prisons and jails than in inpatient hospitals. More than 2 million people living with mental illness are arrested each year; three-fourths of them have co-occurring disorders. Those with serious mental illness are 3 to 6 times more likely to be incarcerated than the general population. Once inside, they stay longer; once released, they are substantially more likely to return.[15,16]

SOLUTIONS TO COMBAT OR MINIMIZE THE IMPACT OF DISPARITIES AND TO MAXIMIZE EQUITY IN COMMUNITY MENTAL HEALTH

Multiple solutions are suggested that will advance equity and diminish disparities in community mental health, and improve the lot of those living with mental illness. By committing to battle stigma, maximize funding, enhance workforce development, and improve services that will support patients along their recovery trajectory, significant progress in the effectiveness of community mental health can be made.

Education is a Key Factor in Diminishing Stigma and Facilitating Advocacy

A variety of models have been used in antistigma campaigns:

1. Protest: more exuberant campaigns that garner attention of decision-makers (eg, striking on the capital steps);
2. Education: campaigns that seek to increase one's understanding related to issues, often with a variety of media approaches (eg, meeting with legislators and disseminating pamphlets or fact sheets);
3. Contact: presentations and interactions involving those whose lives have been affected by the topic at hand (eg, consumers, peers, and family members sitting with law enforcement officers teaching them crisis intervention training techniques).

A plethora of national organizations exist that support education and advocacy—Mental Health America, NAMI, and the Treatment Advocacy Center, to name a few. Federal agencies also exist that provide education, and that fund educational opportunities, including the Substance Abuse and Mental Health Services Administration, the National Institutes of Health, and the National Institutes of Mental Health. Professional organizations also offer education and stigma reduction programs, including the American Psychiatric Association (APA), the National Council for Behavioral Health, the National Association of State Mental Health Program Directors, and the National Association of County Behavioral Health and Developmental Disabilities Directors. Additionally, the Substance Abuse and Mental Health Services Administration is funding "serious mental illness advisor," which is administered by the APA, involving multiple mental health organizations who advise callers about mental health care resources.

Maximizing funding in all arenas is paramount. Strategies include lobbying the federal government to prioritize mental health research and expanding Medicaid (presently 33 states and Washington, DC, have officially expanded Medicaid, and Utah, Idaho, and Nebraska voters have approved moving forward with official expansion). Revising Medicare payments to reflect true provider costs and incentivizing innovative (effective) mental health care would encourage providers to engage more willingly and effectively with people living with mental illness. If salaries and benefits are comparable with other medical specialties, more medical students might choose psychiatry as their profession. It would be helpful if states would take the initiative to improve the quality of mental health care provided by state agencies, in lieu of judicial battles that are costly, and typically end with dramatic decrees and federal court monitoring.

Prevention services prove helpful in minimizing the impact of mental illness on the lives of patients, and can expedite access to services. The APA Foundation offers a program called "Typical or Troubled" that educates sentinels in school systems (ie, teachers, coaches) on how to identify children and adolescents who might be presenting with signs and symptoms of mental illness. Teaching pediatricians about the need to inquire about ACEs could make them sentinels for at-risk pediatric populations. Expansion of crisis lines (hot lines, which deal with acute emergencies; warm lines, which deal with subclinical issues that might put patients at risk) might mitigate suicide risk. Posting the National Suicide Prevention Line number (1-800-273-TALK (8255)) in all health care facilities would offer a venue for receiving support and intervention. States around the country are developing gun control laws known as red flag laws, that allow families to petition courts to temporarily remove firearms from those who present a danger to themselves or others. Assisted outpatient treatment is used in several states to ensure that people living with mental illness who are at risk of relapse and who have not actively chosen to follow their treatment plan are closely monitored and supported within the context of a court order to comply with their treatment. Certainly, education of pregnant women (and those trying to get pregnant) about the importance of cessation of tobacco, alcohol, and drugs would be helpful in decreasing the impact of these substances on the fetus and the mother. Consistent screening of post partum women for depression could play an important role in enhancing both maternal and infant health.

Workforce development is key to addressing disparities in community mental health. Broadening the concept of the work force has proven to be a conundrum for some, with the APA opposed to psychologists being given prescribing privileges. Beyond that, expanding the use of advanced nurse practitioners and physician assistants might expand the numbers of patients in community mental health who can be assessed and treated. The inclusion of social workers on the treatment team to provide referrals, intercede with social determinants, and act as sentinels will also prove helpful. Local, regional, state, and federal recruitment and retention strategies should be developed. The use of the National Health Service Corps, where mental health providers work in underserved areas for multiple years to pay off their student loans is gaining momentum. As mentioned in the Maximizing Funding section, establishing employee compensation that is commensurate with the education and the responsibility of the community mental health provider would certainly entice more into the field. In addition, to increasing numbers of providers it is imperative that the diversity of mental health care providers is expanded, and that health care providers receive training that allows them to gain expertise in providing culturally competent trauma-informed care. Expanding the workforce (and hence access) with regard to training and the use of peer specialists is playing an impressive role in many systems of care.[17] Several national action plans have been developed to expand the workforce[18,19]; investment by consumers and families, communities, and state and federal governments is imperative if these plans are to succeed.

Improving access is key to combating disparities in community mental health. A variety of innovative services are developing that facilitate more effective, efficient, and prompt responses to those living with mental illness. In addition to improving the number of health care providers as noted elsewhere in this article, offering different means of access can be helpful. The development of the integrated care model (primary care/mental health care being provided in 1 site) has been shown to be effective in patients receiving assessments and care in a more timely fashion.[20] The use of telemedicine can enhance geographic access.[21] Emergency rooms are now beginning to work together in systems, creating psychiatric bed registers so that collectively providers can know, in the moment, about bed use. Development of psychiatric urgent care centers has proven effective in taking pressure off of emergency rooms, and are helpful in initiating treatment more rapidly. The use of mobile crisis units and full-fidelity Assertive Community Treatment teams sends professionals out to the patients, which can expedite assessment and care. In addition, training law enforcement on how to handle mental health crises with crisis intervention training has been shown to mitigate incarceration; drug courts, mental health courts, and veterans courts are all diverting people with mental illness away from the criminal justice system back to their community mental health system.[15] Finally, it is imperative that community mental health patients be welcomed into whichever door they choose (or are asked) to come through. Staff should be trained on maintaining a warm, helpful, problem solving attitude; calm and comforting milieus should be the goal, and culturally competent trauma-informed treatment offered (including, if needed, interpreters).[22]

Resources

Often, people living with mental illness who come for community mental health treatment are those who are struggling to find resources beyond those specifically related to mental health. Any capacity to support housing first policies, shelters, or sober living situations will prove helpful. Patients are often unemployed or underemployed, and without financial resources. Although many community mental health treatment centers are not in the job-finding business, developing relationships with vocational rehabilitation or drop-in centers/clubs that offer vocational support can prove invaluable. Offering assistance with Supplemental Securities Income or Social Security Disability Income applications for those who are disabled and unable to work can send a powerful message of care, concern, and support, establish the underpinnings of a trusting relationship, which in turn might help with adherence.

SUMMARY

Given the historical underpinnings of stigma and discrimination, it is not surprising that disparities exist in community mental health. Huge numbers of Americans have diagnosable mental illness, but less than one-half (or worse for some ethnicities) are able or willing to access care. Limited federal and insurance funding can inhibit the capacity of a system of care to provide quality services. Undercompensated mental health services keep salaries and benefits low, which affects the numbers of providers who will choose to do this kind of work (again, limiting access). Emergency rooms are packed, and the number of inpatient hospital beds are dwindling. Patients unable to access care decompensate and often end up homeless and or in the criminal justice system.

To mitigate these disparities, community stigma about mental illness must be battled, federal, state, local and research funding must improve, recruitment and retention strategies for competent mental health staff must be created, and models of innovative services should be evaluated for efficacy, put in place, and sustained.

DISCLOSURE

The author has nothing to disclose.

REFERENCES

1. Institute of medicine (US) committee on understanding and eliminating racial and ethnic disparities in health care. In: Smedley BD, Stith AY, Nelson AR, editors. Unequal treatment: confronting racial and ethnic disparities in health care. Washington, DC: National Academies Press; 2003. Available at: https://www.ncbi.nlm.nih.gov/books/NBK220352. Accessed January 10, 2020.
2. Porter R. Madness: a brief history. New York: Oxford University Press; 2002.
3. Feldman JM. History of community psychiatry. In: McQuistion HL, Sowers WE, Ranz JM, et al, editors. Handbook of community psychiatry. New York: Springer Science & Business Media, LLC; 2012. p. 11–20 [Chapter 2].
4. Social Solutions. Top 5 barriers to mental healthcare access. Social Solutions. Available at: https://www.socialsolutions.com. Accessed January 4, 2020.
5. Corrigan PW, Watson AC. Understanding the impact of stigma on people with mental illness. World Psychiatry 2002;1:16–20.
6. Everett A, Sowers WE, McQuistion HL. Financing of community behavioral health services. In: McQuistion HL, Sowers WE, Ranz JM, et al, editors. Handbook of community psychiatry. New York: Springer Science & Business Media, LLC; 2012. p. 45–60 [Chapter: 5].
7. National Institutes of Mental Health. Culture, race and ethnicity, a supplement to (1999) Mental Health: a report of the Surgeon General. Office of the Surgeon General/Center for Mental Health Services/National Institutes of Mental Health. 2001. Available at: https://www.ncbi.nim.nih.gov/books/NBK44243. Accessed January 1, 2019.
8. Goldenberg M. How increased fundraising and research dollars for mental health can save lives. 2016. Available at: https://huffpost/entry/how-increased-fundraising. Accessed January 5, 2020.
9. US Department of Health and Human Services. Estimations of funding for various research, conditions and disease categories. Bethesda, MD: US Department of Health and Human Services; 2020. Available at: https://wwwreport.NIH.gov/categorical.spending.aspx. Accessed April 2, 2020.

10. Mental Health America. Prevention and early intervention in Mental Health. 2016. Available at: https://www.mhanational.org/issues/Prevention-and-early-intervention-mental-health-consequences-failing-our-children. Accessed January 4, 2020.

11. Lutterman T, Shaw R, Fisher W, et al. Mental health information: statistics. National Institutes on Mental Health. Available at: https://www.nimh.nih.gov/index.shtml. Accessed December 26, 2019.

12. Heinssen RK, Goldstein AB, Azrin ST. Evidence-based treatment for first episode psychoses: components of coordinated special care. National Institutes of Health. Available at: https://www.nimh.nih.gov/health/topics/schizophrenia/raise. Accessed December 23, 2019.

13. Molfenter T. Reducing appointment no-shows: going from theory to practice. National Institutes of Health. 2013. Available at: https://www.ncbi.nim.nih.gov/pmc/articles/PMC39622671/. Accessed March 30, 2020.

14. Mental Health America. Cultural competence. Mental Health America. Available at: https://www.mhanational.Org/issues/culturalcompetence. Accessed January 5, 2020.

15. Committee on Psychiatry and the Community (Group for the Advancement of Psychiatry). People with mental illness in the criminal justice system: answering a cry for help. Washington, DC: American Psychiatric Association Publishers; 2016.

16. US Department of Justice. Law enforcement response to the mental health crisis. US Department of Justice. Available at: https://cops.usdoj.gov/html/dispatch. Accessed January 12, 2020.

17. Mental Health America. Peer services. Mental Health America. Available at: https://www.mhanational.org/peerservices. Accessed January 15, 2020.

18. Annapolis Coalition of Behavioral Health Workforce. The Annapolis framework for workforce planning in behavioral health. Annapolis Coalition of Behavioral Health Workforce. 2018. Available at: www.annapoliscoalition.com. Accessed January 5, 2020.

19. Hogan MA, Morris JA, Daniels AS, et al. An action plan for behavioral workforce development. Rockville (MD): SAMHSA/HHS; 2007.

20. National Institutes of Mental Health. Integrated care. National Institutes of Mental Health. Available at: https://www.nimh.nih.gov/health/topics/integrated-care/index.shtml. Accessed March 25, 2020.

21. Yellowlees P, Shore JH. Telepsychiatry and health technologies. Washington, DC: American Psychiatric Association Publishers; 2018.

22. Wik A, Hollen V, Beck AJ. Developing a behavioral health workforce. National Association of State Mental Health Program Directors. Available at: https://www.nasmhpd.org. Accessed 04 January 2020.

23. National Alliance on Mental Illness. Mental health by the numbers. National Alliance on Mental Illness. Available at: https://www.nami.org. Accessed December 26, 2019.

24. Centers for Disease Control and Prevention. Mental health: data and publications. Centers for Disease Control and Prevention. Available at: https://www.cdc.gov/mentalhealth/datapubications/index.htm. Accessed January 3, 2020.

25. Weill TP. Insufficient dollars and qualified personnel to meet United States mental health needs. J Nerv Ment Dis 2015;203:233–40.

26. Substance Abuse and Mental Health Services Administration. Workforce. Substance Abuse and Mental Health Services Administration. Available at: https://www.samhsa.gov/workforce. Accessed January 2, 2020.

27. Substance Abuse and Mental Health Services Administration. Core competencies for integrated behavioral health and primary care. Substance Abuse and Mental Health Services Administration. Available at: https://www.integration.samhsa.gov/core-competencies-for-integrated-care. Accessed December 29, 2019.
28. World Economic Forum. The cost of mental disorders. World Economic Forum. 2019. Available at: https://www.weforum.org/agenda/2019/01/. Accessed January 6, 2020.
29. Block J. Shortage of psychiatrists only getting worse. Psychiatry Advisor. Available at: https://www.psychiatryadvisor.com/home/practice-management/shortages-of-psychiatrists-only-getting-worse/. Accessed March 29, 2020.
30. Merritt Hawkins. Psychiatry: the silent shortage. Merritt Hawkins. Available at: https://www.Merritt.Hawkins.com/Uploadedfiles/mhawhitepaper_psychiatrypdf?campaignid. Accessed March 29, 2020.
31. American Hospital Association. The state of the behavioral health workforce: a literature review. American Hospital Association. 2016. Available at: https://www.aha.org/system/files/hpoe/ReportsHPOE/2016/aha_Behavioral_FINAL.pdf. Accessed March 28, 2020.
32. National Council for Behavioral Health. The psychiatric shortage: causes and solutions. National Council for Behavioral Health. 2017. Available at: https://www.thenationalcouncil.org/wp-content/uploads/2017/03/Psychiatric-Shortage_National- Council-.pdf?daf=375ateTbd56. Accessed January 6, 2020.
33. Moran M. Psychiatry match numbers continue to climb. Psychiatric News 2019. Available at: https://psychnews.psychiatryonline.org/doi/10.1176/appi.pn.2019.4b24. Accessed January 3, 2020.
34. Glover A, Orlowski JM. The nation's physician workforce and future challenges. Am J Med Sci 2016;351:11–9.
35. Rao S, How PC, Ton H. Education, training, and recruitment of a diverse workforce in psychiatry. Psychiatr Ann 2018;48:143–8.
36. American Hospital Association. Increasing access to behavioral health advances values for patients, providers and communities. American Hospital Association. 2019. Available at: https://www.aha.org/system/files/media/file/2019/05/aha-trendwatch-behavioral-health-2019.pdf. Accessed January 4, 2020.
37. Bishop TF, Press MJ, Keyhani S. Acceptance of insurance by psychiatrists and the implications for access to mental health care. JAMA 2014;71:176–81.
38. McGuire TG, Alegria M, Cook BL, et al. Implementing the Institute of Medicine definition of disparities: an application to mental health care. Health Serv Res 2006;41:1979–2005.
39. McGuire TG, Miranda J. New evidence regarding racial and ethnic disparities in mental health: policy implications. Health Aff 2018;32:22.
40. Wells KB, Klap R, Koike A, et al. Ethnic disparities in unmet need for alcoholism, drug use, and mental health care. Am J Psychiatry 2001;158:2027–32.
41. Substance Abuse and Mental Health Services Administration. Racial/ethnic differences in mental health service. Substance Abuse and Mental Health Services Administration. Available at: https://store.samhsa.gov/product/Racial-Ethnic-Differences-in- Mental-Health-Service-Use-Amongst- Adults/sma15-4906. Accessed January 2, 2020.
42. American Hospital Association. Trend in psychiatric inpatient capacity, United States and each state 1970- 2014. American Hospital Association. Available at: https://www.nasmhpd.org/sites/defaut/files/TAC.paper_. Accessed January 4, 2020.

43. Torrey EF, Entsminger E, Geller J, et al. The shortage of public hospital beds for mentally ill persons. Arlington (VA): Treatment Advocacy Center; 2008.

44. Alderman M, Dasgupta A, Henderson R, et al. Tackling the mental health crisis in emergency departments. Health Aff blog 2018. Available at: https://www.healthaffairs.org/do/10.1377/hblog2018123.22248/full. Accessed January 4, 2020.

45. US Department of Health and Human Services. Mental health: myths and facts. US Department of Health and Human Services. Available at: https://www.mentalhealth.gov. Accessed January 3, 2020.

Two Systems, One Population:
Achieving Equity in Mental Healthcare for Criminal Justice and Marginalized Populations

Sarah Y. Vinson, MD[a,b,*], Timothy T. Coffey, MS[c],
Nicole Jackson, DSW[b], Courtney L. McMickens, MD, MPH, MHS[d,1],
Brian McGregor, PhD[e], Steven Leifman, JD[f]

KEYWORDS

- Criminal justice system reform • Interdisciplinary collaboration
- Criminal justice system diversion

KEY POINTS

- Given the over-representation of those with mental illness in the criminal justice system, interdisciplinary collaboration between the criminal justice and mental health care systems is key to addressing mental health inequities.
- Unmet mental health needs of marginalized populations drive criminal justice system inequities.
- The prevailing approach to those with mental illness in the criminal justice system worsens mental health outcomes in this vulnerable population.
- Opportunities for interdisciplinary collaboration, service linkage, diversion, and intervention exist at every step of criminal justice system involvement.

[a] Morehouse School of Medicine, Atlanta, GA, USA; [b] Lorio Forensics, 675 Seminole Avenue Northeast Unit T-03, Atlanta, GA 30307, USA; [c] Eleventh Judicial Circuit of Florida, Criminal Mental Health Project 1351 Northwest 12th Street Room 226, Miami, FL 33125, USA; [d] Lorio Forensics, Atlanta, GA, USA; [e] Kennedy Satcher Center for Mental Health Equity, Satcher Health Leadership Institute, Morehouse School of Medicine, 720 Westview Drive Southwest, Atlanta, GA 30310, USA; [f] Miami-Dade County Court Eleventh Judicial Circuit of Florida, 1351 Northwest 12th Street Room 617, Miami, FL 33125, USA
[1] Present address: 601 Pembroke Road #4261, Greensboro, NC 27404.
* Corresponding author. Lorio Forensics, 675 Seminole Avenue Northeast Unit T-03, Atlanta, GA 30307.
E-mail address: svinson@msm.edu

Psychiatr Clin N Am 43 (2020) 525–538
https://doi.org/10.1016/j.psc.2020.05.006
0193-953X/20/© 2020 Elsevier Inc. All rights reserved.

Abbreviations	
CIT	Crisis Intervention Team
CMHP	Criminal Mental Health Project
LBGTQ+	Lesbian, gay, bisexual, transgender, queer
MD-FAC	Miami-Dade Forensic Alternative Center
SMI	Serious mental illness

INTRODUCTION

Marginalized populations failed by the housing, child welfare, educational, and employment systems are at higher risk for mental illness; however, far too often, the mental health system, be it private or public, is not readily accessible, culturally responsive, or a reliable source of effective interventions for them. When untreated mental illness results in behaviors that do not conform to societal expectations, people from these populations are disproportionately funneled into the criminal justice system. Unlike the school system that expels them, the housing system that evicts them, the employment system that never hires or readily fires them, and the mental health system that denies or delays their treatment for a myriad of reasons, the gates of the criminal justice system are always open. As such, it is a system where the marginalized and those living with mental illness are greatly over-represented.

In the United States, the country with the world's leading incarceration rate,[1] the criminal justice system's approach to these populations has grave implications for population mental health. **Box 1** includes information about mass incarceration and the criminalization of people with mental illness.

Modern-era studies estimate the number of persons diagnosed with serious mental illness (SMI) in correctional facilities is more than 3 times the number in hospitals.[2] How is it that the care of such a large population has been ceded to the criminal justice system without a strident outcry from the mental health professional community? Tragically, the house of medicine is often guilty of marginalization, too, particularly of those with criminal justice system involvement. Understanding the issues of mass incarceration, criminal justice inequities, and the criminalization of those with mental illness is imperative for any leader striving to address mental health inequities.

This article provides a multidisciplinary examination of the bidirectional interplay of mental health and criminal justice inequities, the historical context for the prevailing extant approaches to correctional mental health treatment, and a case-based exploration of potential programmatic approaches to addressing these inequities across systems.

Box 1
Mass incarceration and the criminalization of people with mental illness

- The criminal justice system has increased by more than 500% in the past 40 years.[1]

- Approximately 6.7 million people were under some form of correctional control by the end of 2015.[46]

- There were 2.2 million physically incarcerated in jails and federal, state, or local prisons in 2016.[47,48]

- Of federal prison inmates, state prison inmates, and local jail inmates, 44.8%, 56.2%, and 64.2%, respectively, reported impairment over the previous year owing to a mental health problem.[49]

- Two-thirds of males and three-quarters of females in previous studies of juvenile offender detention facilities were found to meet criteria for at least 1 mental health disorder.[50,51]

Data from Refs [1,46–51].

MENTAL HEALTH INEQUITIES DRIVING CRIMINAL JUSTICE SYSTEM INEQUITIES

Mental illness disparately impacts the vulnerable in the larger society including, but not limited to, people of color, lesbian, gay, bisexual, transgender, queer (LGBTQ+) populations, and the poor. These factors interact as well. For example, institutionalized racism perpetuates the overrepresentation of African American and Latinx populations among poor, homeless and low socioeconomic status groups, which are less likely to receive timely and appropriate mental health services.[3–5] Contributing factors to this unmet need include an underfunded and inefficient behavioral health safety net.[6] Additionally, given the importance of cultural considerations in behavioral health care delivery,[7] the gross underrepresentation of providers from these groups has negative implications for care.[8,9] It is no coincidence that these 2 racial groups are some of the most adversely impacted by criminal justice disparities: the black–white state imprisonment disparity is 5.1 to 1.0, and the Latinx–white disparity is 1.6 to 1.0.[10]

Although not all members of the LGBTQ+ community have the same experiences, as a group, they are more than twice as likely to experience mental health problems than the general population and are at higher risk for suicide attempts.[11] Sexual minority women are disproportionately incarcerated, especially sexual minority females of color, in both the juvenile and adult justice systems. This may be the result of persistent structural biases or the influence of a pathway from juvenile detention to adult incarceration, or both.[12]

Individuals with traumatic exposures are also over-represented in the criminal justice system, which often limits rather than alleviates mental wellness and recovery. Economically disadvantaged communities are overexposed to psychological trauma in the form of chronic victimization and related stressors, increasing the risk of mental illness. This is true across racial/ethnic groups.[13] Further, socioeconomically disadvantaged individuals with mental health problems are vulnerable to becoming entrenched in the criminal justice system for several reasons:

- They are highly visible to law enforcement because they are over-represented among homeless populations and may be experiencing the disorganizing effects of their illness.[14]
- Compared with those not diagnosed with a mental illness, they are more likely to be arrested for the same behavior, tend to stay in jail and prison longer, and are less likely to be approved for probation or parole than others charged with similar offenses.[15,16]
- Upon release, they are more likely to be rearrested, particularly those with co-occurring illnesses, compared with those not diagnosed with a mental illness.[16–18]
- Recidivism often occurs owing to technical violations of probation and parole conditions rather than new charges, which may be due to social determinants of health, such as housing insecurity and transportation challenges.[17–19]

Accessible, effective, evidence-based treatment along with the necessary support services in community mental health settings may help decrease the over-representation of individuals with mental and substance use disorders in the criminal justice system; however, societal resource allocation decisions indicate that making this the norm is not a priority. State spending on mental health funding for children and adults was cut by close to $2 billion between 2009 and 2011.[20] The impact of these significant reductions is decreased resources for community members, an increase in emergency department visits and inpatient hospitalizations, deepening poverty, and early death. Conversely, corrections budgets increased by a striking 145% between 1986 and 2001.[20]

These sociocultural issues provide a context in which mental illness has been criminalized in part owing to unavailable or insufficient mental health care services. They created pathways into jails and prisons, weakened community ties, and fed intractable cycles of recidivism. Although it is true that targeting criminogenic risk factors, such as family and marital dysfunction, antisocial cognition, and school and work problems, are needed to disrupt these cycles, decriminalizing mental illness will require a realignment of the fractured mental health system, an alignment that ensures the needs of all individuals and communities, including those most vulnerable to trauma and marginalization, are met.

CRIMINAL JUSTICE INEQUITIES DRIVING MENTAL HEALTH INEQUITIES
Mass Incarceration as a Social Determinant of Health

Although studies suggest that there may be beneficial health effects during incarceration attributed to access to health care and reduced exposure to violence and substances, these data vary, and benefits are often short lived. In general, incarceration has an overall negative impact on individual well-being.[21] Increasingly, involvement in the justice system in itself has been associated with negative health consequences. For most individuals involved in the justice system, incarceration is a fraction of their adult lives. The average individual who is imprisoned spends 6 times as long living their adult lives after incarceration.[21] This is a period of significant health risk owing to a lack of continuity of health care, as well as barriers to employment, housing, and social connection.[22]

Involvement in the justice system has a significant impact on the health of those directly involved through incarceration, probation, and parole, as well as on families and whole communities. The Centers for Disease Control and Prevention define social determinants of health as "complex, integrated, and overlapping social structures and economic systems that are responsible for most health inequities."[23] Furthermore, the World Health Organization notes that "social determinants of health are shaped by the distribution of money, power, and resources throughout local communities, nations, and the world."[24] Although not routinely characterized as such, by these definitions individual criminal justice system involvement as well as membership, be it demographic or physical, in a community over-represented in the criminal justice system certainly qualifies.

Individual, Family, and Community Impacts

By design, incarceration undermines basic human needs for mental well-being, including personal agency, safety and security, and access to natural social supports, to name a few. It is no wonder that it is associated with a lifetime prevalence of mood disorders[25] and a greater number of psychosocial problems and more severe symptoms in people with first episode psychosis.[26] Additionally, research demonstrates that even brief periods of incarceration among people with SMI (eg, schizophrenia spectrum disorders, bipolar disorder, and major depressive disorder) are associated with destabilizing, negative outcomes such as disruptions in housing, health care, and critical social supports.[27]

Furthermore, the effects of incarceration often extend to families. In fact, 1 study even linked parental incarceration to child mortality.[28] Several studies have shown an association between parental incarceration and behavioral issues,[29] and parental incarceration has been specifically associated with depression, anxiety, asthma, and obesity in children.[30] Other studies have shown that women with incarcerated partners have elevated cardiac risk factors.[31]

In disproportionately impacted communities, which are already suffering from community violence, hypersegregation and poverty, the harmful impact of mass incarceration and the constant threat of it takes many forms:

- Felony disenfranchisement (when felony convictions result in the loss of voting rights)
- Chronic unemployment and underemployment
- Poor health care quality and limited access to health care
- Unstable housing
- Food insecurity[32]

HISTORY AND TRENDS IN CORRECTIONAL MENTAL HEALTH TREATMENT

A long-standing tension exists between the criminal justice and mental health systems. Although these institutions were established with specific and distinct intentions, their forced intersection by virtue of their overlapping populations poses the need for strategic coordination. Some argue such coordination is nearly impossible in the absence of major criminal justice system reforms crafted and implemented with the needs of persons with SMI in mind.[33]

The US Department of Justice's stated purpose is the promotion of safety through the prevention and control of crime by implementing appropriate punishments to those deemed guilty of unlawful behaviors. Themes from this charge permeate the justice system's priorities: security, safety, power, and control.[33] Naturally, correctional facilities mirror this approach, as they historically and currently have used strategies to impose control over those who pose a threat, or are perceived to do so, during confinement. Although "law and order" may be an operative method of governing the general population, historical lessons illustrate that it is a drastically flawed, yet repeatedly used means for addressing justice system-involved people with trauma and SMI.

The increase in incarceration rates among individuals with SMIs surged after deinstitutionalization in the 1960s and 1970s, as the federal government reformed state-run psychiatric systems and treatment approaches. This movement thrived on new discoveries with psychotropic medications and increased arguments supporting community-based mental health programs versus long-term treatment facilities.

Although some persons benefited from the reformation, the elimination of long-term treatment facilities was devastating for others, because many previously serviced by residential institutions possessed challenges far beyond what community-based interventions were prepared to tackle. This was a key contributor to the criminalization of those with mental illness,[33] a contention supported by a study finding that between 40,000 and 72,000 of those individuals were later found to be incarcerated.[34] Making matters worse, significant challenges were identified within health care services in jail facilities in the 1970s,[2] with mental health services not regarded as standard failing to be provided.

Consequently, statistics soon revealed that correctional facilities were servicing more persons with a SMI than designated mental health facilities. Credited for exacerbating this epidemic are the "tough on crime policies" promoted in the 1980s and 1990s, which implemented harsher sentences for individuals charged with drug-related offenses.[34] The muted truth was that many of these persons were suffering as a result of their unattended mental illness.

Symptoms of mental illness often produce profound dysfunction of cognitions and behaviors, influencing those who are incarcerated to behave in ways viewed as problematic or defiant, and otherwise punishable.[33] Historically, corrections staff have responded to these behaviors with the use of prolonged periods of isolation, as well as physical and chemical restraints.[35] In the 1990s, supermaximum security, or "supermax," prisons became a popular trend, representing a philosophic shift in the management of problematic inmates from a "dispersion" to a "concentration" approach. The basis of this approach is the belief that prisons will be safer and better controlled upon the removal of "menaces."[36,37]

These supermax correctional facilities promoted social isolation, provided no source of meaningful activity, and prohibited the opportunity for environmental stimulation. Assignments to them were given to "nuisance" prisoners, which often meant those with mental illness.[38] The use of such harsh methods was rooted in pervasive inadequacies in resources, training, treatment options, and effective interventions in correctional facilities.[37] Failure to appreciate these root factors precluded foundational solutions, predisposing the system to ineffective attempts to control the undesired outcomes.

The mismanagement and, in many cases, additional traumatization of individuals with trauma and SMI remains a significant challenge within the criminal justice system; however, some recent approaches have focused on the provision of cost-effective methods to deliver appropriate and quality care within the correctional setting. Even more promising is the emergence of diversionary methods to prevent incarceration in the first place. These programs include mental health courts, community-based mental health treatment programs, and reentry as a continuum of care.[39,40]

PROGRAMMATIC APPROACHES TO ADDRESSING INEQUITIES
The Case for Multisystem Collaboration

Although improving access to community-based care is critical to improving outcomes, it is not enough to prevent unnecessary justice system involvement on its own. Services typically available in the community mental health marketplace tend to be insufficient in scope and intensity to address the complex needs of individuals who experience the most severe and persistent forms of mental illness and are at highest risk for involvement in the justice system and other institutional settings.[41]

Those with SMI, members of marginalized populations, and people with dual diagnoses are over-represented in criminal justice and underserved by the mental health care system, and they face added challenges to accessing, engaging, and complying with treatment. Currently, both the public and private systems of care fall short. Services that do exist tend to be inadequately funded, antiquated, and fragmented. Furthermore, inefficiencies in service delivery are compounded by poor coordination, treatment gaps, and redundancies across the system of care.

Fortunately, there are promising solutions that have been developed as the result of innovative relationships and collaborations at the intersection of the criminal justice and mental health systems:

- Crisis Intervention Teams (CIT) that teach law enforcement officers to better recognize and respond to psychiatric emergencies in the community
- Jail diversion programs and mental health courts that use specialized dockets and provide judicial monitoring of treatment linkages and engagement
- Reentry programs that assist with linkages to treatment and support services upon completion of jail or prison sentences

- Community corrections programs that employ specially trained officers who apply problem-solving strategies to enhance compliance with terms of probation or parole

A Case Study: The Eleventh Judicial Circuit Criminal Mental Health Project

The following is an illustration of a program in operation in Miami-Dade County, Florida, that draws on a variety of problem-solving strategies to decrease demand for mental health services provided in the criminal justice system. The Eleventh Judicial Circuit Criminal Mental Health Project (CMHP) was established in 2000 to divert individuals with SMI or co-occurring SMI and substance use disorders away from the criminal justice system and into comprehensive community-based treatment and supports.

The program operates 2 primary components: prebooking jail diversion consisting of CIT training for law enforcement officers and postbooking jail diversion serving individuals booked into the county jail and awaiting adjudication. In addition, the CMHP offers a variety of overlay services with distinct, but related goals:

- Streamline screening and identification of program participants
- Develop evidence-based community reentry plans to ensure appropriate linkages to community-based treatment and support services
- Improve outcomes among individuals with histories of noncompliance with treatment
- Expedite access to federal and state entitlement benefits

The CMHP provides an effective, cost-efficient solution to a community problem and works by eliminating gaps in services through forging productive and innovative relationships among all stakeholders who have an interest in the welfare and safety of one of our community's most vulnerable populations. **Fig. 1** presents CMHP results since 2008.

Prebooking Jail Diversion: Officer Training and Crisis Intervention Training

The purpose of the CIT training (also known as the Memphis model) is to set a standard of excellence for law enforcement officers with respect to treatment of individuals with mental illness.[42] CIT officers perform regular duty assignment as patrol officers, but are also trained to respond to calls involving mental health crises. Officers receive 40 hours of specialized training in psychiatric diagnoses, suicide

Officers respond to nearly 20K mental health crisis calls per year.	**The number of annual jail bookings has decreased from roughly 118K to 53K in 2018.**	**The average daily population in the county jail has dropped from 7.2k to 4.2k in 2019.**	**Th county has closed an entire jail at a cost-savings to taxpayers of $12 million per year.**

Fig. 1. CMHP results since 2008. (*Courtesy of* T.T. Coffey, Miami, FL. and S. Leifman, JD, Miami FL.)

intervention, substance use disorders, behavioral deescalation techniques, the role of the family in the care of a person with mental illness, mental health and substance abuse laws, and local resources for those in crisis. The training is designed to educate and prepare officers to recognize the signs and symptoms of mental illness, and to respond more effectively and appropriately to individuals in crisis. When appropriate, individuals are assisted in accessing treatment in lieu of being arrested and taken to jail.

To date, the CMHP has provided CIT training to more than 7000 law enforcement officers from all 36 municipalities in Miami-Dade County, as well as Miami-Dade Public Schools and the Department of Corrections and Rehabilitation. **Fig. 2** shows outcomes data illustrating the program's effectiveness.

Postbooking Jail Diversion

A multistep process is used to identify defendants with mental illness who are brought into the jail, starting at the time of booking. The goal is to support community living, reduce maladaptive behaviors, and decrease the chances that individuals will reoffend and reappear in the criminal justice system.

1. All booked defendants are screened for signs and symptoms of mental illnesses by correctional officers using evidence-based screening tools, including the Texas Christian University Drug Screen V[43] and the Ohio Risk Assessment: Community Supervision Tool.[44]
2. Defendants undergo medical screening by health care staff at the jail, which includes additional assessment of psychiatric functioning.
3. Those identified as being in possible psychiatric distress are referred to corrections health services' psychiatric staff for more thorough evaluation.
4. CMHP screens each program participant for mental health and substance use treatment needs, as well as criminogenic risk factors to determine the appropriate level of treatment, support services, and community supervision.
5. A 2-page summary is used to develop an individualized transition plan aimed at decreasing criminal justice recidivism and improved psychiatric outcomes, recovery, and community integration.
6. Upon stabilization, legal charges may be dismissed or modified in accordance with treatment engagement.

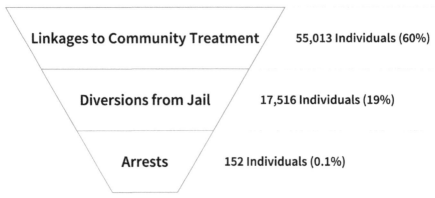

Fig. 2. Outcomes of 91,472 crisis cases to CMHP CIT officers. (*Courtesy of* T.T. Coffey, Miami, FL. and S. Leifman, JD, Miami FL.)

7. Individuals who voluntarily agree to services are assisted with linkages to a comprehensive array of community-based treatment, support, and housing services that are essential for successful community reentry and recovery outcomes.
8. The CMHP uses the Assess, Plan, Identify, and Coordinate model, a nationally recognized best practice model, to provide transition planning for all program participants.[45]

This approach has proven effective:

- Recidivism rates among program participants have decreased from roughly 75% to 20% annually among misdemeanor jail diversion program participants.
- Total jail bookings and days spent in the county jail among felony jail diversion program participants decreased by 59% and 57%, respectively.
- The outcome is a difference of approximately 31,000 fewer days in jail, nearly 84 years of jail bed days.

Forensic Hospital Diversion Program

Since August 2009, the CMHP has overseen the implementation of the Miami-Dade Forensic Alternative Center (MD-FAC), a program designed to divert individuals with mental illnesses who are adjudicated incompetent to proceed to trial from placement in state forensic hospitals to placement in community-based treatment and forensic services. As the number of people with mental illnesses entering the justice system increases, competency restoration has become a significant issue for many states. See **Box 2** for additional information regarding competency to stand trial.

Participants in the MD-FAC program include individuals charged with second- and third-degree felonies who do not have significant histories of violent felony offenses

---

Box 2
Background information regarding competency restoration

- The Fifth Amendment entitles everyone to the right to a fair trial. This means that criminal cases cannot move forward if defendants do not have an appreciation of the nature and potential consequences of the charges filed against them, and/or cannot assist in their own defenses. Defendants who are unable to do these things are deemed "incompetent to stand trial."

- After someone is determined to be incompetent to stand trial, they have to be "restored" to competency before the case moves forward. This can be through legal education and or treatment of whatever condition is prohibiting them from being competent. This process is called "competency restoration."

- The goal of competency restoration, which is often provided in inpatient forensic hospital settings, is not treatment for the purposes of recovery, but treatment to satisfy a legal threshold.

- Once the defendant's competency has been restored, treatment may be discontinued. In cases of charges that do not merit incarceration, not guilty findings, or dropped charges, the person is often released to the community with no additional care.

- Not only are these competency restoration services not conducive to recovery, but they are also incredibly expensive. For example, the state of Florida currently spends 25% of its entire mental health services budget—approximately $212 million annually—for 1652 forensic beds in state mental health treatment facilities serving approximately 4012 individuals.

- Because of the right to a fair trial, competency restoration is an entitlement that states must fund, often at the expense of more effective long-term care in the community.

and are not likely to face incarceration if convicted of their alleged offenses. The community-based treatment provider operating services for the project is responsible for providing a full array of residential treatment and community reentry services, including crisis stabilization, competency restoration, development of community living skills, assistance with community reentry, and community monitoring to ensure ongoing treatment after discharge. The treatment provider also assists individuals in accessing entitlement benefits and other means of economic self-sufficiency to ensure ongoing and timely access to services and supports after reentering the community.

Unlike individuals admitted to state hospitals, individuals served by MD-FAC are not returned to jail upon restoration of competency, thereby decreasing burdens on the jail and eliminating the possibility that a person may decompensate while in jail and require readmission to a state hospital. To date, the project has demonstrated more cost-effective delivery of forensic mental health services, decreased burdens on the county jail in terms of housing and transporting defendants with forensic mental health needs, and more effective community reentry and monitoring of individuals who, historically, have been at high risk for recidivism to the justice system and other acute care settings.

Individuals admitted to the MD-FAC program are identified as ready for discharge from forensic commitment an average of 52 days (35%) sooner than individuals who complete competency restoration services in forensic treatment facilities and spend an average of 31 fewer days (18%) under forensic commitment. The average cost to provide services in the MD-FAC program is roughly 32% less expensive than services provided in state forensic treatment facilities.

Looking Ahead: The Miami Center for Mental Health and Recovery

The CMHP is working with stakeholders from Miami-Dade County, the state of Florida, and a local nonprofit managing entity known as Thriving Mind South Florida on a capital improvement project to develop a first-of-its-kind mental health diversion and treatment facility, which will expand the capacity to divert individuals from the county jail into a seamless continuum of comprehensive community-based treatment programs that leverage local, state, and federal resources.

The purpose of the Miami Center for Mental Health and Recovery is to create a comprehensive and coordinated system of care for individuals with SMIs who are

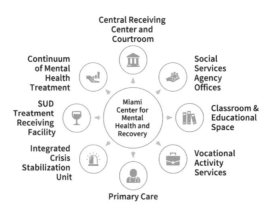

Fig. 3. Components of the Miami Center for Mental Heath and Recovery. SUD, substance use disorder. (*Courtesy of* T.T. Coffey, Miami, FL. and S. Leifman, JD, Miami FL.)

As Clinicians
- Understand the impact of mass incarceration on communities
- Assess for trauma and loss associated with criminal justice system involvement
- Self-assess for personal bias and be intentional in taking a non-judgmental stance

 As Collaborators
- Be intentional about devoting time to forging connections & engaging across disciplines
- Participate in providing CIT trainings
- Be aware of local criminal justice diversion programs and seek out collaboration

 As Administrators
- Examine hiring and patient care policies for discriminatory practices
- Track engagement and outcomes with traditionally under-served populations
- Be intentional about hiring, training and mentoring a representative workforce

 As Advocates
- Engage your local professional organization in matters pertaining to criminal justice reform
- Contact local legislators and indicate interest in being a resource regarding trauma informed care and evidence-based practices
- Inform your professional community by inviting speakers with criminal justice expertise

Fig. 4. Mental health. Clinician approaches to addressing inequities at the intersection of mental health and criminal justice. (*Courtesy of* S.Y. Vinson, MD, Atlanta, GA.)

frequent and costly recidivists to the criminal justice system, the homeless continuum of care, and acute care medical and mental health treatment systems. The building encompasses approximately 181,000 square feet of space and capacity for 208 beds. Operation at the facility will begin in early 2021. See **Fig. 3** for additional information about the facility's offerings.

The CMHP offers the promise of hope and recovery for individuals with SMI that have often been misunderstood and discriminated against. Once engaged in treatment and community support services, individuals can achieve successful recovery, community integration, and reduce their engagement with the criminal justice system.

SUMMARY

A multisystemic problem of this magnitude requires a broad-based interdisciplinary response. A basic understanding of mass incarceration's mental health impacts should be considered foundational knowledge for all public sector mental health professionals. In turn, this understanding could inform approaches to addressing inequities at the intersection of mental health and criminal justice on the clinical, administrative, and community levels. As examples, clinicians can fold assessment for trauma and loss associated with criminal justice system involvement into their patient encounters; and administrators can be intentional about hiring, training, and mentoring a representative workforce. There is work to be done outside of clinical settings as well through intersystem collaboration and advocacy efforts. **Fig. 4** explores how this effort can be approached through these various avenues.

Both patient-centered care and the medical ethics principle of justice demand that mental health providers are not only aware of criminal justice system inequities but are also actively working within and across systems to eliminate them.

DISCLOSURE

Judge S. Leifman and Mr T.T. Coffey are administrators in the Eleventh Judicial Circuit CMHP program discussed in the article. None of the other authors have anything to disclose.

REFERENCES

1. The Sentencing Project. U.S. prison population trends: massive buildup and modest decline. 2019. Available at: Sentencingproject.org. Accessed December 9, 2019.
2. Torrey EF, Kennard AD, Eslinger D, et al. More mentally ill persons are in jails and prisons than hospitals: a survey of the states. 2010. Available at: http://tulare.networkofcare.org/library/final_jails_v_hospitals_study1.pdf. Accessed December 7, 2019.
3. Paradies Y, Ben J, Denson N, et al. Racism as a determinant of health: a systematic review and meta-analysis. PLoS One 2015;10(9):1–48.
4. Jones CJ. Levels of racism: a theoretical framework and a gardner's tale. Am J Public Health 2000;90:1212–5.
5. U.S. Department of Health and Human Services, Substance Abuse and Mental Health Services Administration, Center for Mental Health Services. Mental Health: Culture, Race, and Ethnicity—A Supplement to Mental Health: A Report of the Surgeon General. 2001.
6. McMorrow S, Gates JA, Long SK, et al. Medicaid expansion increased coverage, improved affordability, and reduced psychological distress for low-income parents. Health Aff 2017;36(5):808–18.
7. McGregor B, Belton A, Henry TL, et al. Commentary: improving behavioral health equity through cultural competence training of health care providers. Ethn Dis 2019;(Supp 2):359–64.
8. U.S. Census Bureau. American Community Survey 1-Year PUMS file. 2015. Available at: www.census.gov/programs-surveys/acs/data/pums.html. Accessed December 21, 2019.
9. Duffy FF, West JC, Wilk J, et al. Mental health practitioners and trainees. In: Manderscheid RW, Henderson MJ, editors. Mental health, United States, 2002. DHHS Publication No. SMA 04- 3938. Rockville (MD): U.S. Department of Health and Human Services, Substance Abuse and Mental Health Services Administration, Center for Mental Health Services; 2004. p. 327–68.
10. Sabol WJ, Johnson TL, Caccavale A. Trends in correctional control by race and sex. Washington, DC: Council on Criminal Justice; 2019.
11. Medley G, Lipari RN, Bose J, et al. Sexual orientation and estimates of adult substance use and mental health: results from the 2015 National Survey on Drug Use and Health. NSDUH Data Review. 2016. Available at: http://www.samhsa.gov/data/. Accessed December 21, 2019.
12. Wilson BDM, Jordan SP, Meyer IH, et al. Disproportionality and disparities among sexual minority youth in custody. J Youth Adolesc 2017;46(7):1547–61.
13. Jaggi LJ, Mezuk B, Watkins DC, et al. The relationship between trauma, arrest and incarceration history among black Americans: findings from the national survey of American life. Soc Ment Health 2016;6(3):187–206.
14. Kouyoumdjian FG, Wang R, Mejia-Lancheros C, et al. Interactions between police and persons who experience homelessness and mental illness in Toronto, Canada: findings from a prospective study. Can J Psychiatry 2019;64(10):718–25.
15. U.S. Bureau of Justice Statistics. Mental health problems of prison and jail inmates. NCJ 213600. 2006. Available at: https://www.bjs.gov/content/pub/pdf/mhppji.pdf. Accessed December 8, 2019.
16. Wilson AB, Draine J, Hadley T, et al. Examining the impact of mental illness and substance use on recidivism in a county jail. Int J Law Psychiatry 2011;34:264–8.

17. Feder L. A comparison of the community adjustment of mentally ill offenders with those from general population: an 18 month follow up. Law Hum Behav 1991; 15(5):477–93.

18. Louden JE, Skeem JL, Camp H, et al. Supervising probationers with mental disorder: how do agencies respond to violations? Crim Justice Behav 2008;35(7): 832–47.

19. Baillargeon J, Williams BA, Mellow J, et al. Parole revocation among prison inmates with psychiatric and substance use disorders. Psychiatr Serv 2009; 60(11):1516–21.

20. National Alliance on Mental Illness. State mental health cuts: a national crisis. 2011. Available at: www.nami.org/budgetcuts. Accessed December 9, 2019.

21. Wildeman C, Wang EA. Mass incarceration, public health, and widening inequality in the USA. Lancet 2017;389(10077):1464–74.

22. Lee H, McCormick T, Hicken MT, et al. Racial inequalities in connectedness to imprisoned individuals in the United States. Du Bois Rev 2015;12:269–82.

23. CDC. NCHHSTP social determinants of health. Atlanta (GA): CDC; 2014. Available at: https://www.cdc.gov/nchhstp/socialdeterminants/definitions.html.

24. World Health Organization (WHO). Closing the gap in a generation: health equity through action on the social determinants of health. Final report of the Commission on Social Determinants of Health (CSDH): Geneva. 2008. Available at: https://apps.who.int/iris/bitstream/handle/10665/43943/9789241563703_eng. pdf;jsessionid=FCA63F55FEC0A35EC04F619E133FB6C0?sequence=1.

25. Schnittker J, Massoglia M, Uggen C. Out and down: incarceration. Lancet 2016; 388:1103–14.

26. Ramsay CE, Goulding SM, Broussard B, et al. Prevalence and psychosocial correlates of prior incarcerations in an urban, predominantly African-American sample of hospitalized patients with first-episode psychosis. J Am Acad Psychiatry Law 2011;39(1):57–64.

27. Lowencamp C, VanNostrand M, Holsinger A. The hidden costs of pre-trial detention. Houston (TX): Laura and John Arnold Foundation; 2013.

28. Wildeman C, Anderson SA, Lee H, et al. Parental incarceration and child mortality in Denmark. Am J Public Health 2014;104(3):428–33.

29. Murray J, Farrington DP, Sekol I. Children's antisocial behavior, mental health, drug use, and educational performance after parental incarceration: a systematic review and meta-analysis. Psychol Bull 2012;138(2):175–210.

30. Turney K. Stress proliferation across generations? Examining the relationship between parental incarceration and childhood health. J Health Soc Behav 2014; 55(3):302–19.

31. Lee H, Wildeman C, Wang EA, et al. A heavy burden: the cardiovascular health consequences of having a family member incarcerated. Am J Public Health 2014;104(3):421–7.

32. Legal Action Center. After prison: roadblocks to reentry. a report on state legal barriers facing people with criminal records 2009. Available at: https:// csgjusticecenter.org/nrrc/publications/after-prison-roadblocks-to-reentry-2/. Accessed December 8, 2019.

33. Fellner J. A corrections quandary: mental illness and prison rules. Harv CR-CLL Rev 2006;41:391–411.

34. Travis J, Western B, Redburn FS. The growth of incarceration in the United States: exploring causes and consequences. Washington, DC: The National Academies Press; 2014.

35. Patterson RF. Our part in the revolution of correctional mental health care. J Am Acad Psychiatry Law 2018;46:140–6.
36. Riveland C. Supermax prisons: overview and general considerations. Washington, DC: National Institute of Corrections; 1999.
37. Metzner J, Dvoskin J. An overview of correctional psychiatry. Psychiatr Clin North Am 2006;29:761–72.
38. Glidden B, Rovner L. Requiring the state to justify supermax confinement for mentally ill prisoners: a disability discrimination approach. Denv UL Rev 2012; 90:55–75.
39. Tamburello A, Kaldany H, Dickert J. Correctional mental health administration. Int Rev Psychiatry 2017;29:3–10.
40. Bradley- Engen M, Cuddeback G, Gayman M. Trends in state prison admission of offenders with serious mental illness. Psychiatr Serv 2007;61:1263–5.
41. Leifman S, Coffey T. The sequential intercept model and criminal justice: promoting community alternatives for individuals with serious mental illnesses. In: Griffin PA, Heilbrun K, Mulvey EP, et al, editors. Rethinking mental health legal policy and practice: history and needed reforms. New York: Oxford University Press; 2015. p. 188–216.
42. Dupont R, Cochran S. Police response to mental health emergencies: barriers to change. J Am Acad Psychiatry Law 2000;28:338–44.
43. Fort Worth: Texas Christian University Institute of Behavioral Research. Texas Christian University Drug Screen 5; 2017.
44. Latessa E, Smith P, Lemke R, et al. Creation and validation of the Ohio risk assessment system: final report. Cincinnati (OH): University of Cincinnati, School of Criminal Justice, Center for Criminal Justice Research; 2009.
45. Osher F, Steadman HJ, Barr H. A best practice approach to community re-entry from jails for inmates with co-occurring disorders: the APIC model. Delmar (NY): The National GAINS Center; 2002.
46. U.S. Bureau of Statistics. Correctional populations in the United States, 2015. NCJ 250229 2016. Available at: http://www.bjs.gov/index.cfm?ty=pbdetail&iid=5871. Accessed December 8, 2019.
47. U.S. Bureau of Statistics. Prisoners in 2016. NCJ 251149. 2018. Available at: http://www.bjs.gov/index.cfm?ty=pbdetail&iid=6187. Accessed December 8, 2019.
48. U.S. Bureau of Statistics. Jail Inmates in 2016. NCJ 251210. 2018. Available at: http://www.bjs.gov/index.cfm?ty=pbdetail&iid=6186. Accessed December 8, 2019.
49. Bureau of Justice Statistics. Mental health problems of prison and jail inmates (DOJ Publication No. NCJ 213600). Washington, DC. 2006. Available at: www.bjs.gov/content/pub/pdf/mhppji.pdf.
50. Wasserman GA, McReynolds LS, Lucas CP, et al. The voice DISC-IV with incarcerated male youths: prevalence of disorder. J Am Acad Child Adolesc Psychiatry 2002;41:314–21.
51. Huizinga D, Loeber R, Thornberry T, et al. Co-occurrence of delinquency and other problem behaviors. Washington, DC: Office of Juvenile Justice and Delinquency Prevention; 2000.

Consumer and Family Perspectives to Achieve Mental Health Equity

Chirlane I. McCray

KEYWORDS

- Consumer • Family • Equity • Recovery • ThriveNYC • New York City

KEY POINTS

- Consumers and their families offer an integral source of knowledge for mental health providers, and the inclusion of that knowledge in care planning and delivery is essential to build mental health equity.
- The advocacy efforts of consumers and families have improved mental health care across several dimensions, including deinstitutionalization, the acceptance and proliferation of recovery-oriented care, and reductions in population-level mental health stigma.
- To leverage public policy to build mental health equity, New York City has launched ThriveNYC, the nation's largest municipal-level mental health program. ThriveNYC prioritizes the voices of consumers and families at all levels of care.

Broad and equitable access to mental health treatment has greatly improved in the United States in recent years. The treatment parity for mental health services established by the Affordable Care Act, Medicaid expansion in most states, and acceptance of mental health as a critical component of the health care system all have helped reduce disparities in access and outcomes by race, gender, socioeconomic status, and sexual orientation.[1]

Despite these gains, large disparities remain,[2] including between people of color and white people.[3] White Americans are diagnosed and treated for mental health conditions at higher rates than black or Latinx Americans,[4] despite evidence that black and Latinx Americans demonstrate higher levels of psychological distress.[5] When black and Latinx individuals do receive mental health treatment, they are more likely to be hospitalized or institutionalized than white individuals,[6] indicating an urgent need for appropriate and supportive community-based mental health care systems to serve communities of color.

In addition, women are nearly twice as likely as men to suffer poor mental health outcomes,[7] and black women bear a disproportionate share of diagnoses.[8] Although

181 East End Avenue, #2, New York, NY 10128, USA
E-mail address: Chirlane@mac.com

Psychiatr Clin N Am 43 (2020) 539–554
https://doi.org/10.1016/j.psc.2020.06.003
0193-953X/20/Published by Elsevier Inc.

psych.theclinics.com

women are more likely to disclose symptoms and seek help within the health care system,[9] they are at risk of serious repercussions for doing so. Black women with diagnosed mental illness are nearly twice as likely to lose custody of their children as women without such symptoms.[10] Findings indicate that up to 40% of children with parents who experience symptoms of mental illness also will develop symptoms by age 20.[11]

People who identify as lesbian, gay, bisexual, or transgender (LGBT) are more than twice as likely to be diagnosed with a mental health disorder as heterosexual-identified individuals.[12] Lack of access to LGBT-affirming mental health care is a barrier for many people; findings suggest that transgender persons are 2.4 times as likely to report unmet mental health needs as their cisgender counterparts.[13] This disparity is exacerbated by race, with black and Latinx LGBT individuals demonstrating poorer mental health outcomes than white LGBT individuals.[14]

These disparities are far-reaching. Recent research has identified that experiencing injustice in the forms of racism,[15] sexism,[16] and homophobia[17] is broadly associated with poorer mental health outcomes. In order to close these gaps, mental health equity must become and remain a guiding principle for health care providers and policymakers. Unconscious racial bias in clinical practice also is well documented,[18] and clinicians have the professional and moral responsibility to identify and unlearn biases that do unintended harm to patients of color and patients from marginalized communities. Policymakers can prioritize equity through the strategic allocation of funding and health care resources. The communities that experience the greatest burdens—black and brown communities and poor communities—should receive the necessary resources to adequately address mental health needs at the individual and population levels. As demonstrated in New York City and nationally, health policy rooted in and oriented toward equity can and should be cultivated and operationalized at all levels of government.

This article argues that clinicians and policymakers can prioritize mental health equity through the recognition and inclusion of consumer and family perspectives in their work. These perspectives often have been excluded from health care research and policy with harmful consequences. In summary, this article will (1) introduce consumer and family perspectives and describe their connections to mental health equity; (2) share a portion of the lead author's personal mental health journey as a consumer, family member, and advocate; (3) briefly review the empirical literature that supports the inclusion of these perspectives into clinical care and policymaking; (4) identify how consumers and families have contributed to the mental health field; (5) present 2 examples of how consumer and family perspectives have been operationalized to improve population- and individual-level mental health care; and (6) describe several strategies to integrate these perspectives into public health practice as part of a broad equity agenda.

DEFINING CONSUMER AND FAMILY PERSPECTIVES

A first step to integrating consumer and family perspectives into mental health treatment and policy is to arrive at a clear definition for research and practice. First, it is important to identify mental health as distinct from mental illness. "Mental health" refers to personal and social well-being through which individuals realize their own abilities and are able to cope with routine life stresses to work productively and fruitfully within their communities and is distinct from "mental illness," which refers to diagnosable health conditions associated with distress or impaired functioning that are characterized by alterations in thinking, mood, or behavior.

Several definitions of "consumer" have been put forward in professional mental health and psychiatry.[19] These fields have debated who is considered a consumer and how "consumers" are qualitatively different from "survivors" or "former patients."[20] I define consumers as individuals who use mental health services, assuming that their care and engagement with services is voluntary. In this context, "family" denotes the support systems—families of origin and families of choice—that aid consumers as they enter care and progress toward recovery.

Although mental health "patients" are often thought of as passive recipients of treatment, consumers and families are active participants in both the planning and the delivery of care. As the foremost experts in their own experiences,[21] consumers have agency to make decisions about their recovery. Health care providers can listen to their voices and take their wishes seriously. Crediting the expertise held by consumers—especially consumers from marginalized communities—is an important first step toward closing gaps in mental health equity. Evidence indicates that individuals who feel validated and heard by their mental health providers experience better outcomes than those who do not feel that they have agency in their own recovery.[22] Incorporating consumer and family perspectives routinely into care will afford providers a fuller picture of consumers and facilitate treatment of the whole person, not just a person's symptoms.

PERSONAL TO POLITICAL: MY JOURNEY AS A CONSUMER, FAMILY MEMBER, AND ADVOCATE

I feel called to my work as a mental health advocate because of my own lived experience and the experiences of people I love. When I was a girl, my family was one of two black families living in our neighborhood in western Massachusetts. I was the only black student in all of my classes from kindergarten through high school. I often was bullied, taunted, and shamed, which was witnessed and ignored by my teachers. Although some students and teachers were kind and friendly, the discrimination I endured left me sad and anxious, feelings that stayed with me throughout my youth.

I could not express those feelings at home. My father was a World War II veteran whose family emigrated from the South during the Great Migration, and my mother was the daughter of immigrants from Barbados. Together, they worked hard to provide my siblings and me with opportunities they never had, and their sacrifices helped me become the woman I am today. But they were not communicative people. They were not verbal about their emotions and were often withdrawn. We knew they loved us, but we did not discuss our feelings as a family, especially not negative ones.

Looking back, I believe my parents' behavior stemmed from the difficulties they had experienced in their own lives, which they had no way to process. My own feelings were an early indicator of developing mental health challenges. But it was a long journey to identifying and interpreting what was happening to me, and I carried that baggage into adulthood.

In my early adult years, I worked a short time as a full-time, freelance writer in New York City, a stressful job filled with financial uncertainty, quick deadlines, and challenging assignments. When *Essence* magazine asked me to write a piece called, "How to Know When You Need Therapy," I found myself unable to complete the assignment or do any other work. I had never been to therapy and was not in touch with my own mental health needs.

As it turns out, the assignment was timely. This was a difficult period for me. For the first time in my life, I lacked drive and direction and didn't know how to fix myself. I was smoking marijuana regularly and, although I did not believe I was physically addicted, I found it difficult to stop. A helpful friend connected me to a social worker, who over time helped me process the emotions that led me to smoke and better manage my life. It was my first experience with therapy and the first time I was forced to consider my mental health.

Many years later, when my own children were young, my mother was diagnosed with multiple myeloma. I went through a period of extreme stress as I attempted to care for my children and coordinate my mother's care, all while working full time. I was exhausted and physically ill. It took the help of an empathic and thoughtful gastroenterologist to help me understand that I was exhibiting signs of anxiety and depression. He presented the option for me to temporarily treat it with medication. I took the medication but discontinued as soon as I was able, although I continued to struggle.

When my daughter revealed her own struggles with depression, anxiety, and addiction, I felt helpless. She was 18 years old and therefore expected to navigate her own care, but her illness made that nearly impossible. She could hardly get out of bed, let alone find an appropriate and affordable provider who could connect with her experiences as a young biracial student.

I felt at a loss to help her. There was no established series of steps to take. I didn't understand the vocabulary; it often sounded like a foreign language. I didn't know what type of provider to look for. My husband and I had to trust the recommendations of people we did not know well. We had to make major decisions based on faith. Thankfully, we eventually found enough of what we were looking for. Our daughter managed her recovery, engaged in work to help other young people who were going through similar struggles, and successfully graduated from college.

Although I did not recognize it until recently, while working again with a therapist, it is clear to me that I have suffered from some level of anxiety and depression most of my life. I am on a lifelong journey to better manage my condition and am taking proactive steps to manage and improve my own mental health.

None of my experiences—as a child, as an adult, or as a mother—are unique. Unspoken, untreated mental illness and substance use disorders are common, as are the pain and confusion that come with them. I consider myself fortunate to eventually have found care as an adult, even during the period when I had no health insurance. I also was fortunate to find resources to support my daughter. Many without such resources suffer a long time, with great negative impact on their quality of life.

The other half of my personal journey with mental health is political. Although I was not aware of it as a child, I grew up during a time of significant change in mental health policy, the age of deinstitutionalization. I was 9 years old when President Kennedy signed the Community Mental Health Act into law just weeks before his death. The new law directed states to close their psychiatric hospitals and open community mental health centers in their places. The vision and spirit of the law were admirable—that consumers could receive humane and comprehensive mental health care while being bolstered by the support of their families and communities.

But this vision was never fully realized. Without the federal support necessary, many states closed their institutions without replacing them with community-based services. More than half of the community health centers proposed by the legislation never opened. Some people with mental health needs were supported by families and loved ones (with great financial burden), but others had no support system. With nowhere to go, many people ended up on the streets or in shelters, and innumerable others were unjustly detained in jails and prisons. The effects of this failure linger and have hardened into our nation's entwined crises of homelessness, suicide, and overdose. City leaders across the country are grappling with these challenges.

That is why, as First Lady of New York City, I am committed to improving mental health at the population level and building a community mental health infrastructure that is humane and just. With that goal in mind, I have worked closely with New York City's elected leaders and public health officials to develop and launch Thrive-NYC, an overarching policy framework to incorporate mental health equity across all aspects of urban governance.[23] As the City began to refine its approach to mental health, I joined New York City's public health leadership on an 11-month information-gathering tour. Through listening sessions, town halls, and focus groups, New York City's public health leadership and I spoke with community service providers, faith leaders, educators, family members, and people with lived experience dealing with mental health challenges, as well as traditional health experts, researchers, and clinicians.

These conversations helped to identify critical needs and gaps in New York City's mental health services. I heard from immigrants and people of color about their struggles to find culturally competent clinicians. I heard from educators who witness how trauma prevents the children in their classrooms from learning. I heard from faith leaders and social service providers in low-income neighborhoods who saw the need in their communities but lacked the tools and resources to help. I heard about the expense and accessibility barriers to mental health services that prevent so many individuals from receiving care. Nearly everyone with whom I spoke shared their experiences with the overwhelming stigma around mental illness and mental health treatment in the United States.

These problems are inextricable from the racial, economic, and social inequities that harm so many members of our society. Mental health cannot be improved without addressing and fostering mental health equity. Since we first embarked on our information-gathering tour, elevating the voices of consumers and family members has remained essential to ThriveNYC's work.

With ThriveNYC, we have an opportunity in New York City to meet the mental health needs of all of our diverse communities. By honoring the knowledge to be gained from consumers and families, we are building a mental health platform grounded in equity—growing community mental health from the bottom up. Our approach has the potential to benefit not just New York City but also cities across the country.

CONSUMER AND FAMILY PERSPECTIVES: SCIENCE AND JUSTICE

A growing body of research indicates that mental health outcomes improve when providers listen to and take seriously the perspectives of consumers and families as part of care planning and delivery.[19] This active engagement strengthens the relationship between consumers and providers,[24] which in turn helps to rebuild trust between consumers and the mental health system. Increased trust consequently may lead to increased retention in care, which is associated with improved outcomes.[25] Through an equity lens, rebuilding trust between the mental health care system and communities systematically excluded from or harmed by that system—such as black and brown communities and the LGBT community—is critical if we are to improve population-level mental health.[26]

There are several highly effective strategies used to engage consumers and families in care. These include the integration of peers (ie, persons with lived experience) into professionalized treatment teams[27]; strategic coordination to break down barriers between consumers and their primary care providers, mental health providers, and other specialist health care and social service providers[28]; and task-sharing to leverage community-based support networks to deliver care outside of traditional psychiatric or psychotherapeutic settings.[29,30] In the current era of evidence-based health policy, providers and policymakers must acknowledge emerging evidence in support of the integration of consumer and family perspectives into care.

The use of peer supports empowers consumers to identify outside the role of "patient"; the empathic perspective of the peer builds trust with the consumer and offers a model for recovery and support along the way.[31] Research into the use of peers in mental health care teams indicates that the integration of peer support is feasible in a wide range of community- and hospital-based settings.[32] Evaluations of peer support models have demonstrated that the use of peers is associated with improved mental health and social outcomes, including reduced hospitalizations,[33] reduced criminal justice involvement and substance use,[34] and improved consumer quality of life.[35] In addition, peer models are an effective means to engage consumers who historically may have faced discrimination within or exclusion from the health care system, including people of color and the LGBT community.[36,37]

Strategic care coordination engages the expertise of a consumer's full care team—including providers, peer supports, and consumers and their families—in a shared decision-making process about mental health care.[38] Care coordination and shared decision making restore agency to consumers in determining their mental health care, allowing them to proceed as they are comfortable.[39] This practice also individualizes care to meet consumers' unique needs[40] and is associated with improved social outcomes in a mental health recovery framework.[41,42]

As a means of integrating peers, consumers, families, and care coordination beyond the health care system, task-sharing is a novel approach to care that engages community members and care workers who are not mental health professionals in community-based mental health care.[43] Although task-sharing initially was designed to expand access to care in low-resource jurisdictions, the principles of task-sharing fit neatly within a mental health equity frame.[44] Evaluations of task-sharing models have linked the practice to improved mental health outcomes, including symptom reduction and increased quality of life.[45] Evidence also indicates that task-sharing can reduce health care costs and increase the efficiency of care delivery.[46]

As the empirical evidence demonstrates, peer support, strategic care coordination, and task-sharing are effective models for integrating and amplifying the voices of consumers and families. In addition to the scientific case, there also is a strong moral case to be made: including the perspectives of consumers and families is the right thing to do. Feelings of exclusion and alienation can drive individuals out of care,[47] even when care is accessible and available. For communities that historically have been marginalized from mental health care, inclusion is critical to rebuilding trust in health professionals and the larger mental health system. If practitioners and policymakers take mental health equity seriously, the perspectives of consumers and families must be front and center in their work.

NOTING THE ACHIEVEMENTS OF CONSUMERS AND FAMILIES

Although consumer and family voices only recently have been elevated in mental health care, consumers and families have achieved much to build mental health equity in the last half-century. Most notably, the passage of the Community Mental Health Act marked the end of the era of institutionalization and codified into law the notion that mental health consumers have rights.[19] Empowerment is fundamental to this policy framework.[48] Despite the limitations of deinstitutionalization in the United States, this thinking represented a major sea of change. Before the consumer movement, the notion that individuals could actively determine their own mental health outcomes was considered preposterous by the medical establishment.[49] Viewing this shift through the lens of mental health equity, it becomes clear how race, class, gender, and sexuality are linked to a mental health framework that prioritizes consumer agency.

In tandem with the consumer movement in mental health, the field was transformed by the reorientation from "cure" to "recovery." The shift toward recovery-oriented care has helped consumers and providers identify new metrics to understand wellness beyond traditional diagnostic criteria.[50] Providers and consumers began to understand mental health as more than a confluence of symptoms and diagnoses. Rather, mental health is continually in process and can be managed toward outcomes chosen by the consumer. Recovery is self-defined in collaboration with families and care teams. Although "cure" may be the goal for some consumers, it is not the goal for all consumers.[51] It took decades of advocacy for mental health providers to respect consumer agency and let recovery be defined and directed by the individual.

The sum of these paradigm shifts has been reduced stigma, shame, and silence around mental health in US culture. Although stigma persists and is pernicious, consumers and their families are now able to come out of the shadows and share their stories.[52] This is not without cost, and it would be dangerous to understate the personal risks involved with sharing one's mental health story. But when knit together, these small personal acts of bravery help normalize mental health and are tremendously important to both our culture and the medical field. Only by joining personal storytelling with rigorous science can we continue not just to reduce but also to undo and unlearn stigma.

CONSUMER AND FAMILY PERSPECTIVES IN PRACTICE: IMPROVING POPULATION- AND INDIVIDUAL-LEVEL CARE

Given the overwhelming scientific and moral justification for the recognition and inclusion of consumer and family perspectives in treatment, it is important to detail concrete examples in which consumers and their families have come together to improve mental health care and outcomes. The National Alliance on Mental Illness (NAMI), a grassroots advocacy group founded by and comprising consumers and families, and Fountain House, a treatment center that prioritizes the agency of consumers in their own care, are 2 models that demonstrate how a consumer- and family-first framework for mental health can be put into practice. These examples work across the spectrum of mental health, from policy and advocacy to treatment and clinical care, to prioritize consumers and families at the population and individual levels.

NAMI was founded in 1979 by family members of mental health consumers who believed that they and their loved ones had a right to be active agents in their own mental health treatment.[53] It was built on 5 core beliefs about mental health: (1) mental illness should be considered a chronic health condition like any other; (2) mental illness is the fault of no one, not the consumer nor their families; (3) family is an integral piece of any successful treatment plan; (4) laypersons without formal medical or mental health training have valuable knowledge and experience and can organize to advocate for their own and their loved ones' needs; and (5) society has an obligation to provide care and treatment to individuals with mental health needs.[54] Since its founding, the organization has grown into the largest mental health advocacy group in the United States, with representation in all 50 states, Washington DC, and Puerto Rico.

In addition to federal and state advocacy, the organization develops and disseminates education, antistigma materials, and programming tailored for various audiences, such as students, clinicians, and family members. NAMI also operates a toll-free, peer-support hotline for mental health consumers and family members to obtain information, share their experiences with a nonjudgmental peer, and identify routes of care tailored for their needs.[54] Evaluations of NAMI's programming indicate that its antistigma education materials have a demonstrable impact on knowledge production and stigma reduction.[55] NAMI's family treatment advocacy training improves family members' abilities to advocate for their loved ones' care and navigate the health care system,[56] and its family peer-support course improves coping and reduces stress for primary caregivers.[57] In addition to serving as a critical resource for consumers, families, providers, and policymakers, NAMI demonstrates the collective power of consumers and families in helping to transform the health care and mental health treatment systems.

Fountain House, a community mental health recovery program founded in New York City in 1948,[58] is an individual-level correlate to the population-level education and advocacy work conducted by NAMI. Today, Fountain House is both a treatment facility and a model of care grounded in community inclusion that welcomes consumers not as patients but as "members" of the Fountain House "clubhouse."[59] Members at Fountain House are involved in all aspects of care for themselves and other members. Residents run the facility as part of community engagement and workforce skill-building. The model is one of a "working community"; in providing for themselves and the other members, a community is built and individuals are drawn out of the social isolation that so often accompanies mental illness.[60]

The model prioritizes the expressed needs of clubhouse members as the necessary components of individuals' plans for care. At Fountain House, treatment plans are generated bottom-up from the member to the community to the clinician, rather than top-down from the clinician to the individual patient. The clubhouse model has been implemented in more than 300 programs worldwide, and evaluations indicate that the community and social support offered helps to build member self-efficacy, self-confidence, and practical skills for moving into recovery.[61,62] Taken together, NAMI and Fountain House represent the success and engagement in care that comes when consumer and family perspectives are prioritized by policymakers and the health care system.

ThriveNYC: PUBLIC POLICY TO IMPROVE MENTAL HEALTH EQUITY

To build mental health equity at the broadest level in New York City, the City of New York launched ThriveNYC in 2015.[23] ThriveNYC seeks to institutionalize the population-level advocacy and individual-level service delivery innovations pioneered by organizations like NAMI and Fountain House within municipal government. The portfolio constitutes the nation's largest municipal-level mental health policy platform, an investment of approximately $250 million per year over the last 4 years. ThriveNYC's work prioritizes equity and inclusion, builds the evidence base for innovation, and is motivated by 6 foundational principles:

1. *Change the culture*: Changing who is involved in mental health care delivery by undoing stigma and putting a new face on recovery.
2. *Act early*: Changing when intervention occurs by investing in the mental health of the youngest New Yorkers to build a healthier future.
3. *Close treatment gaps*: Changing where care is delivered by ensuring that all New Yorkers have access to the mental health services that work for them.
4. *Partner with communities*: Changing how care is delivered by bolstering the mental health care infrastructure in nontraditional settings so that New Yorkers feel comfortable accessing services in their communities.

5. *Use data better*: Changing what data are collected and used by centering marginalized communities and focusing on mental health equity.
6. *Strengthen government's ability to lead*: Changing why governments invest in community mental health by bringing new voices into policymaking.

These principles guide and inform 4 programmatic goals, around which a series of interlocking initiatives are organized: (1) eliminate barriers to care; (2) reach those with the highest need; (3) strengthen crisis prevention and response; and (4) develop resiliency for the youngest New Yorkers. No matter how broad or how narrow its scope, each ThriveNYC initiative works toward mental health equity.

For example, as evidence indicates that early intervention is crucial to lifelong mental health,[63] we have introduced a social-emotional learning curriculum into New York City prekindergarten classrooms. This curriculum teaches and cultivates children's social, emotional, and behavioral regulation skills to intervene early and prevent mental health issues before they start. The curriculum includes supports for parents and caregivers to break cycles of intergenerational mental health stigma and trauma.

We know that task-sharing can help reduce disparities in access to mental health services.[43] Through the Connections to Care initiative, we have integrated mental health supports into places where people already spend their time—such as faith-based organizations and community centers—and are training nonspecialist community leaders and service providers that individuals trust to recognize and take action to support their neighbors', clients', and community's mental health. We are taking seriously where treatment services are located through our place-based supports, an important strategy to build up community-based mental health care.[64] More people are accessing treatment in their neighborhood and in nontraditional ways, with new direct care services in senior centers, homeless shelters, schools, and community-based organizations.

Access to information is critical for individuals in crisis or who are struggling with their own or a loved one's mental health.[65] To ensure that access to information, support, and referrals is available whenever and wherever people need it, we have launched NYC Well, a call, text, and chat hotline that provides crisis counseling, referrals to mental health and social services, peer support, short-term telephonic psychotherapy, and individualized follow-up upon request 24 hours per day, 7 days per week, 365 days per year, with interpretation available for more than 200 languages. In addition, to meet the unique and urgent mental health needs of victims of crime,[66] we have implemented the Crime Victim Assistance Program, which integrates victim advocate and supportive counseling services in all police precincts in New York City. Providers follow up with victims to assist with safety planning, employment advocacy, and connections to therapy that can help victims take back their lives after an experience of trauma. These are just several examples, and ThriveNYC continues to grow. For policymakers and providers who wish to take up this charge in their own work, a selection of the ThriveNYC portfolio and ThriveNYC-aligned initiatives is presented in **Table 1**.

In New York City, we aim to lead by example. The ThriveNYC approach is adaptable for any community and has been implemented successfully in jurisdictions worldwide. For example, in 2017, the Mayor of London launched ThriveLDN, a citywide framework for mental health equity in London that builds directly on ThriveNYC and uses public policy to meet the unique mental health needs of Londoners.[67,68] In Stockholm, the ThriveNYC model was adapted as Mind Shift, a cross-sector initiative that brings together a diverse range of stakeholders to develop a policy platform for mental health

Table 1
ThriveNYC select initiatives

Key Principle	Equity Goal	Description	Select Initiatives
Change the culture	Change who is involved in care delivery	Undoing mental health stigma so that all New Yorkers feel comfortable to engage in care	*Weekend of Faith:* Annually convening over 2000 faith communities in New York City to hold conversations about mental health and learn how to educate congregations about available supports and leverage existing faith-based resources *Peer workforce development:* Cultivating the peer workforce across New York City's mental health infrastructure, including training and integration into crisis response services *Mental Health First Aid:* Training lay New Yorkers to recognize symptoms, feel comfortable talking about mental health, and refer people to appropriate community services. By normalizing conversations about mental health, Mental Health First Aid breaks down stigma
Act early	Change when intervention occurs	Investing in the mental health of the youngest New Yorkers to build a healthier future	*Social-emotional learning:* Incorporating social, emotional, and behavioral regulation skills into New York City's prekindergarten curriculum at schools citywide to prevent adverse mental health outcomes before they start, with additional support and training available for parents and caregivers *School-based restorative justice:* Using restorative justice in lieu of traditional punitive school sanctions to engage youth in needed emotional support and break the school-to-prison pipeline by avoiding criminal justice contact for students whenever possible
Close treatment gaps	Change where care is delivered	Ensuring that all New Yorkers have access to the mental health care that works for them	*Place-based supports:* Integrating peers and mental health professionals into community settings to reach populations at high need and high risk outside of the traditional health care infrastructure. Settings include schools to reach children and youth and intervene early; senior centers to reach older adults, whose needs may have gone neglected; family shelters to engage children and parents at extraordinarily high risk of adverse outcomes, including newborns; and adult shelters to reach and support individuals with complex care needs *NYC Well:* Building a 24/7 hotline to provide crisis counseling, referrals to mental health and social services, appointment scheduling and introductions to community-based providers, peer support, short-term telephonic psychotherapy, and follow-up upon request. Services are available by call, text, or chat to deliver information and support to anyone, anywhere, anytime, with interpretation available for more than 200 languages

Partner with communities	Change how care is delivered	Building out the mental health care infrastructure in community-based and nontraditional locations so that New Yorkers feel comfortable accessing care in their communities	*Connections to Care*: Integrating mental health support into community-based organizations outside of the traditional mental health infrastructure (eg, daycare centers, job training programs, shelters) to build task-sharing partnerships with mental health providers. Staff are trained and coached on how to screen and engage clients around mental health and offer direct support or refer appropriately *Crime Victim Assistance Program*: Embedding trained mental health advocates into all police precincts across New York City to support victims of crime, including domestic violence, at the earliest appropriate opportunity. Advocates provide supportive counseling, safety planning, liaisons to employers and landlords for accommodations, assistance with applications to victim compensation funds, and connection to individual or group therapy
Use data better	Change what data are collected	Shaping the data we collect and using it to improve service delivery	*Data dashboard*: ThriveNYC will report nearly 100 outcome measures on a quarterly basis, testing the efficacy of its dozens of programs in making real change in the lives of New Yorkers
Strengthen government's ability to lead	Change why government invests in community mental health	Bring new voices into mental health policy to ensure that policies meet the needs of communities	*NYC Mental Health Council*: Formalizing and sustaining a body of representatives from >20 New York City government agencies to engage ThriveNYC principles in all aspects of their work

framed in prevention rather than treatment.[69] In addition, through the Cities Thrive Coalition, we have called on municipal governments across the United States to take up mental health equity as a major policy goal. New York City regularly hosts the Cities Thrive Coalition summit, and, as of 2019, more than 200 cities and counties have pledged their support to implement best practices and develop new strategies to improve population-level mental health.

In addition to fulfilling the obligation municipal governments have to support the well-being of their residents, city leaders across the globe also are recognizing the opportunity inherent in this work. Mental health touches all aspects of urban policy and governance, from housing and homelessness to criminal justice and education. By enacting strategies to improve mental health and advance mental health equity and bringing more voices to the table than ever before, local governments can accelerate broader social and economic progress.

SUMMARY

This article has emphasized the importance of consumer and family perspectives to individual-level care and population health policy. Mental health is deeply personal, and my own experiences called me to work as an advocate. Similarly, consumers, families, and policymakers are informed by their own experiences as they develop solutions and navigate systems of care. The concrete strategies detailed here are empirically grounded and tightly focused on equity, as our work must be if we are going to bring mental health to all New Yorkers. ThriveNYC and Cities Thrive represent large steps forward in our collective progress toward mental health equity, but they are only the first steps. The gaps in mental health equity were borne over generations, and our work will not undo that harm overnight.

Reflecting on my own journey, I think about how my family and I might have benefited from the community-based and community-oriented programs and policies that we are implementing in New York City. As a young girl, I was involved with the Girls' Club, the Y, and a local community center—the kinds of places where ThriveNYC is reaching New Yorkers through Connections to Care. During my school days, a social-emotional learning curriculum could have helped me better understand and cope constructively with my feelings. When I was robbed at gunpoint as a young woman, the Crime Victim Assistance Program could have helped me navigate the justice system and process the trauma of that experience. There also could have been a parent component to my daughter's program that could have helped me to better understand and support her journey.

One of the driving ideas behind ThriveNYC is that many untapped opportunities exist to reach people with mental health support. Local governments can and must do more to seize those opportunities. Empowering consumers and family members with knowledge, while undoing stigma across our culture, will help individuals use their voices to engage in recovery without fear or shame. By treating mental health as a human right, as New York City is doing with ThriveNYC, policymakers can fundamentally alter the mental health landscape. The vision for community-based care is achievable. Mental health equity is achievable. But it will take all of us—policymakers, practitioners, consumers, and family members—working together to build the just world we deserve.

ACKNOWLEDGMENTS

I want to thank Hillary Kunins for her expertise and guidance in developing this article along with Bennett Allen, whose support helped streamline this piece and finalize it.

DISCLOSURE

The author have nothing to disclose.

REFERENCES

1. Adepoju OE, Preston MA, Gonzales G. Health care disparities in the post-Affordable Care Act era. Am J Public Health 2015;105(Suppl 5):S665–7.
2. National Academies of Sciences, Engineering, and Medicine. In: Baciu A, Negussie Y, Geller A, et al, editors. Communities in action: pathways to health equity. Washington, DC: National Academies Press (US); 2017. p. 2. The State of Health Disparities in the United States. Available at: https://www.ncbi.nlm.nih.gov/books/NBK425844/.
3. McGuire TG, Miranda J. New evidence regarding racial and ethnic disparities in mental health: policy implications. Health Aff 2008;27(2):393–403.
4. Breslau J, Kendler KS, Su M, et al. Lifetime risk and persistence of psychiatric disorders across ethnic groups in the United States. Psychol Med 2005;35(3):317–27.
5. U.S. Department of Health and Human Services. Mental health: culture, race, and ethnicity-a supplement to mental health: a report of the surgeon general. Rockville (MD): U.S. Department of Health and Human Services, Substance Abuse and Mental Health Services Administration, Center for Mental Health Services; 2001.
6. Snowden LR, Cheung FK. Use of inpatient mental health services by members of ethnic minority groups. Am Psychol 1990;45(3):347–55.
7. Weissman MM, Olfson M. Depression in women: implications for health care research. Science 1995;269:799.
8. Miranda J, Green BL. The need for mental health services research focusing on poor young women. J Ment Health Policy Econ 1999;2(2):73–80.
9. Yu S. Uncovering the hidden impacts of inequality on mental health: a global study. Transl Psychiatry 2018;8(1):98.
10. Harp KLH, Oser CB. Factors associated with two types of child custody loss among a sample of African American mothers: a novel approach. Soc Sci Res 2016;60:283–96.
11. Beardslee WR, Versage EM, Gladstone TR. Children of affectively ill parents: a review of the past 10 years. J Am Acad Child Adolesc Psychiatry 1998;37(11):1134–41.
12. Semlyen J, King M, Varney J, et al. Sexual orientation and symptoms of common mental disorder or low wellbeing: combined meta-analysis of 12 UK population health surveys. BMC Psychiatry 2016;16:67.
13. Steele LS, Daley A, Curling D, et al. LGBT identity, untreated depression, and unmet need for mental health services by sexual minority women and trans-identified people. J Womens Health 2017;26(2):116–27.
14. Daniel H, Butkus R. Lesbian, gay, bisexual, and transgender health disparities: executive summary of a policy position paper from the American College of Physicians. Ann Intern Med 2015;163(2):135–7.
15. Paradies Y, Ben J, Denson N, et al. Racism as a determinant of health: a systematic review and meta-analysis. PLoS One 2015;10(9):e0138511.
16. Watson LB, Marszalek JM, Dispenza F, et al. Understanding the relationships among white and African American women's sexual objectification experiences, physical safety anxiety, and psychological distress. Sex Roles 2015;72(3–4):91–104.

17. Meyer IH. Prejudice, social stress, and mental health in lesbian, gay, and bisexual populations: conceptual issues and research evidence. Psychol Bull 2003; 129(5):674–97.

18. Merino Y, Adams L, Hall WJ. Implicit bias and mental health professionals: priorities and directions for research. Psychiatr Serv 2018;69(6):723–5.

19. Tomes N. The patient as a policy factor: a historical case study of the consumer/survivor movement in mental health. Health Aff 2006;25(3):720–9.

20. Sharfstein SS, Dickerson FB. Psychiatry and the consumer movement. Health Aff 2006;25(3):734–6.

21. Tambuyzer E, Pieters G, Van Audenhove C. Patient involvement in mental health care: one size does not fit all. Health Expect 2014;17(1):138–50.

22. Wong EC, Collins RL, Breslau J, et al. Associations between provider communication and personal recovery outcomes. BMC Psychiatry 2019;19(1):102.

23. Belkin G, McCray C. ThriveNYC: delivering on mental health. Am J Public Health 2019;109(S3):S156–63.

24. Marshall SL, Oades LG, Crowe TP. Mental health consumers' perceptions of receiving recovery-focused services. J Eval Clin Pract 2009;15(4):654–9.

25. Dixon LB, Holoshitz Y, Nossel I. Treatment engagement of individuals experiencing mental illness: review and update. World Psychiatry 2016;15(1):13–20.

26. Priebe S, Matanov A, Schor R, et al. Good practice in mental health care for socially marginalised groups in Europe: a qualitative study of expert views in 14 countries. BMC Public Health 2012;12:248.

27. Marill MC. Beyond twelve steps, peer-supported mental health care. Health Aff 2019;38(6):896–901.

28. Patel V, Belkin GS, Chockalingam A, et al. Grand challenges: integrating mental health services into priority health care platforms. PLoS Med 2013;10(5): e1001448.

29. Castillo EG, Ijadi-Maghsoodi R, Shadravan S, et al. Community interventions to promote mental health and social equity. Curr Psychiatry Rep 2019;21(5):35.

30. Grant KL, Simmons MB, Davey CG. Three nontraditional approaches to improving the capacity, accessibility, and quality of mental health services: an overview. Psychiatr Serv 2018;69(5):508–16.

31. Mead S, Hilton D, Curtis L. Peer support: a theoretical perspective. Psychiatr Rehabil J 2001;25(2):134–41.

32. Puschner B, Repper J, Mahlke C, et al. Using peer support in developing empowering mental health services (UPSIDES): background, rationale and methodology. Ann Glob Health 2019;85(1):53.

33. Sledge WH, Lawless M, Sells D, et al. Effectiveness of peer support in reducing readmissions of persons with multiple psychiatric hospitalizations. Psychiatr Serv 2011;62(5):541–4.

34. Rowe M, Bellamy C, Baranoski M, et al. A peer-support, group intervention to reduce substance use and criminality among persons with severe mental illness. Psychiatr Serv 2007;58(7):955–61.

35. Fuhr DC, Salisbury TT, De Silva MJ, et al. Effectiveness of peer-delivered interventions for severe mental illness and depression on clinical and psychosocial outcomes: a systematic review and meta-analysis. Soc Psychiatry Psychiatr Epidemiol 2014;49(11):1691–702.

36. Tondora J, O'Connell M, Miller R, et al. A clinical trial of peer-based culturally responsive person-centered care for psychosis for African Americans and Latinos. Clin Trials 2010;7(4):368–79.

37. Logie CH, Lacombe-Duncan A, Lee-Foon N, et al. It's for us newcomers, LGBTQ persons, and HIV-positive persons. You feel free to be": a qualitative study exploring social support group participation among African and Caribbean lesbian, gay, bisexual and transgender newcomers and refugees in Toronto, Canada. BMC Int Health Hum Rights 2016;16(1):18.
38. Fukui S, Matthias MS, Salyers MP. Core domains of shared decision-making during psychiatric visits: scientific and preference-based discussions. Adm Policy Ment Health 2015;42(1):40–6.
39. Shidhaye R, Lund C, Chisholm D. Closing the treatment gap for mental, neurological and substance use disorders by strengthening existing health care platforms: strategies for delivery and integration of evidence-based interventions. Int J Ment Health Syst 2015;9:40.
40. Morant N, Kaminskiy E, Ramon S. Shared decision making for psychiatric medication management: beyond the micro-social. Health Expect 2016;19(5):1002–14.
41. Slade M. Implementing shared decision making in routine mental health care. World Psychiatry 2017;16(2):146–53.
42. Wakefield P, Read S, Firth W, et al. Clients' perceptions of outcome following contact with a community mental health team. J Ment Health 1998;7(4):375–84.
43. Raviola G, Naslund JA, Smith SL, et al. Innovative models in mental health delivery systems: task sharing care with non-specialist providers to close the mental health treatment gap. Curr Psychiatry Rep 2019;21(6):44.
44. Hoeft TJ, Fortney JC, Patel V, et al. Task-sharing approaches to improve mental health care in rural and other low-resource settings: a systematic review. J Rural Health 2018;34(1):48–62.
45. Javadi D, Feldhaus I, Mancuso A, et al. Applying systems thinking to task shifting for mental health using lay providers: a review of the evidence. Glob Ment Health (Camb) 2017;4:e14.
46. Seidman G, Atun R. Does task shifting yield cost savings and improve efficiency for health systems? A systematic review of evidence from low-income and middle-income countries. Hum Resour Health 2017;15(1):29.
47. Henderson C, Evans-Lacko S, Thornicroft G. Mental illness stigma, help seeking, and public health programs. Am J Public Health 2013;103(5):777–80.
48. Chamberlain J. The ex-patient's movement: where we've been and where we're going. J Mind Behav 1999;11(2–4):323–36.
49. Mclean AH. From ex-patient alternatives to consumer options: consequences of consumerism for psychiatric consumers and the ex-patient movement. Int J Health Serv 2000;30(4):821–47.
50. Davidson L. The recovery movement: implications for mental health care and enabling people to participate fully in life. Health Aff 2016;35(6):1091–7.
51. Noiseux S, St-Cyr Tribble D, Leclerc C, et al. Developing a model of recovery in mental health. BMC Health Serv Res 2009;9:73.
52. Mannarini S, Rossi A. Assessing mental illness stigma: a complex issue. Front Psychol 2019;9:2722.
53. Phillips K. Mental illness is not anyone's fault: a review of NAMI, the National Alliance on Mental Illness. J Consumer Health on the Internet 2020;24(1):75–81.
54. Hatfield AB. The national alliance for the mentally ill: a decade later. Community Ment Health J 1991;27(2):95–103.
55. Corrigan PW, Rafacz JD, Hautamaki J, et al. Changing stigmatizing perceptions and recollections about mental illness: the effects of NAMI's in our own voice. Community Ment Health J 2010;46(5):517–22.

56. Brister T, Cavaleri MA, Olin SS, et al. An evaluation of the NAMI Basics program. J Child Fam Stud 2012;21:439–42.
57. Dixon LB, Lucksted A, Medoff DR, et al. Outcomes of a randomized study of a peer-taught Family-to-Family Education Program for mental illness. Psychiatr Serv 2011;62(6):591–7.
58. Goertzel V, Beard JH, Pilnick S. Fountain house foundation: case study of an ex-patient's club. J Soc Issues 1960;16(2):54–61.
59. Norman C. The Fountain House movement, an alternative rehabilitation model for people with mental health problems, members' descriptions of what works. Scand J Caring Sci 2006;20(2):184–92.
60. Karlsson M. Introduction to mental health clubhouses: how the Fountain House clubhouse became an international model. Int J Self Help Self Care 2013; 7(1):7–18.
61. Chen FP, Oh H. Staff views on member participation in a mental health clubhouse. Health Soc Care Community 2019;27(3):788–96.
62. Prince JD, Mora O, Schonebaum AD. Willingness to ask for help among persons with severe mental illness: call for research. Community Ment Health J 2019; 55(2):249–56.
63. Membride H. Mental health: early intervention and prevention in children and young people. Br J Nurs 2016;25(10):552–4, 556–7.
64. Thornicroft G, Deb T, Henderson C. Community mental health care worldwide: current status and further developments. World Psychiatry 2016;15(3):276–86.
65. Gould MS, Munfakh JL, Kleinman M, et al. National suicide prevention lifeline: enhancing mental health care for suicidal individuals and other people in crisis. Suicide Life Threat Behav 2012;42(1):22–35.
66. Kilpatrick DG, Acierno R. Mental health needs of crime victims: epidemiology and outcomes. J Trauma Stress 2003;16(2):119–32.
67. Kousoulis AA, Goldie I. Mapping mental health priorities in London with real-world data. Lancet Psychiatry 2017;4(10):e24.
68. Mayor of London. ThriveLDN: towards healthier, happier lives. London: Greater London Authority; 2017.
69. Mind Shift. Available at: http://www.mindshift.health/about/. Accessed March 4, 2020.

Training Psychiatrists to Achieve Mental Health Equity

Donna M. Sudak, MD[a],*, Sandra M. DeJong, MD, MSc[b],
Brigitte Bailey, MD[c], Robert M. Rohrbaugh, MD[d]

KEYWORDS

- Advocacy • Mental health equity • Structural competency • ACGME requirement
- Health disparities

KEY POINTS

- Psychiatric diagnosis and treatment of marginalized groups contributes to mental health inequity.
- Recruiting practices to improve diversity in the mental health workforce have been insufficient.
- Educational initiatives in cultural and structural competency may improve mental health equity.
- Child and adolescent psychiatry training is embedded in an underfunded system that needs reform to achieve mental health equity.

The history of inequity in mental health care cannot be separated from racism, homophobia, and other biases in the treatment of multiple marginalized groups. For example, in 1838, William Goodell noted in his review of the American slave code an advertisement from *the Charleston Mercury* soliciting the purchase of slaves who had physical illnesses to be bought by medical institutions to be used for education or experiments after being deemed incurable.[1] In an attempt to correct such past wrongs, efforts have been made to understand and characterize various minority groups for educational purposes. In addition to running the risk of stereotyping, these

[a] Drexel-Tower Health Psychiatry, Drexel University, 219 Broad Street, Fifth Floor #506, Philadelphia, PA 19107, USA; [b] Harvard Medical School, Cambridge Health Alliance, 1493 Cambridge Street, Cambridge, MA 02139, USA; [c] Child and Adolescent Psychiatry, Department of Psychiatry and Behavioral Sciences, University of Texas Health San Antonio, 7703 Floyd Curl Drive MC 7792, San Antonio, TX 78229, USA; [d] Yale School of Medicine, 300 George Street, Suite 901, New Haven, CT 06437, USA
* Corresponding author.
E-mail address: ds42@drexel.edu
Twitter: @DonnaSudak (D.M.S.)

Psychiatr Clin N Am 43 (2020) 555–568
https://doi.org/10.1016/j.psc.2020.05.003
0193-953X/20/© 2020 Elsevier Inc. All rights reserved.

may neglect internal differences between externally perceived categories, as well as between individuals. We have moved from a posture of "cultural competence" to "cultural humility." In writing this article, the authors acknowledge the inability to explicitly describe all aspects of health inequity in diverse groups. Their effort is to capture the historical big picture and a conceptual framework for moving forward.

Historical events such as the Tuskegee Syphilis Study,[2] the wholesale kidnapping of children of American Indian and Native Alaskan families to send them to boarding schools, the designation of homosexuality as an illness until 1973, and the subsequent appropriation of multiple brutal measures to "cure" homosexuality produced heightened suspicion of health care providers by these groups. Psychiatry has a history of characterizing normal behaviors in enslaved and oppressed people as pathologic, which although horrific to consider at present, may have bearing on the perceived "safety" of mental health care. In the 1890s academic psychiatry journals wrote about African Americans as being "psychologically unfit for freedom."[3] Such biased thinking did not stop in the antebellum era and examples have been documented more recently in many racial groups. Rates of diagnosis of schizophrenia in African Americans are known to be higher than in whites, thought to be in part because of underdiagnosing mood disorders.[4] In the 1960s the perception of schizophrenia shifted from an unthreatening illness to an illness characterized by violent behavior in young African American men. African American men were deemed delusional if they were "antiwhite" and the diagnostic criteria in DSM-II changed to include hostility and aggression.[3] African Americans currently receive higher doses of antipsychotic medications in mental health treatment than other groups.[5] Physicians still make clinical decisions based on implicit racial and other stereotypes, such as unconsciously preferring white patients or providing fewer evidence-based treatment recommendations for minority patients.[6]

The lack of equitable mental health care in American Indian and Alaska Natives (AI/AN) stems from structural, diagnostic, and historical factors. First, many traditional AI/AN cultures conceptualize mental illness differently from Western culture. The imposition of a Western worldview about psychiatric illness was made worse by the opening of a federal mental hospital for Native Americans, "The Hiawatha Asylum for Insane Indians," in 1889.[7] This facility was essentially a prison.

At the time of the establishment of this asylum, AI/AN religious and cultural practices were illegal and children of AI/AN were shipped to federal boarding schools, where they were forbidden from engaging in cultural practices and kept in deplorable conditions. As a result, trauma and mistrust pervade AI/AN regarding psychiatry.[8] In the absence of cultural sensitivity and humility, such mistrust in any marginalized person may be misconstrued as paranoia and can result in defensiveness rather than empathic curiosity.

AI/AN are entitled to health benefits by the federal government via the Indian Health Service (IHS) if they are members of recognized tribes. Unfortunately, several issues adversely affect the provision of such care. First, the lack of adherence to treaties has meant that multiple indigenous Americans are uncovered by such benefits. Second, funding for the IHS is woefully inadequate and only extended to tribal members living near a reservation. The IHS per capita spending is less than half the per capita national average for health care and does not include any outpatient mental health services.[9] Furthermore, structural issues significantly affect mental health in the AI/AN community; rates of poverty, high school dropouts, suicide, domestic violence, and substance use disorders are among the highest in any known group.

Health inequity may also occur because of language barriers, which often occurs in the Latinx community due to a lack of Spanish language proficiency in health care providers. Low rates of insurance and reluctance to seek care may relate to concerns about documentation in this community.[10]

RECRUITING PRACTICES THAT CONTRIBUTE TO MENTAL HEALTH INEQUITY

Structural (institutional) racism that prevents minority physicians underrepresented in medicine (URM) from full participation in medicine has existed a hundred years longer than calls to diversify the physician workforce and profoundly affects recruitment and retention of faculty, residents, and medical students.[11]

The history of recruiting URM physicians into the American Medical Association (AMA) and the American Psychiatric Association (APA) further informs our understanding of mental health inequity. The year 1847 was significant in that the AMA was founded and David Jones Peck, the first African American graduate of an American medical school, received his MD from Rush Medical School. In 1854 John Van Surly DeGrasse was the first African American admitted to a US Medical Society in Massachusetts. The Medical Society of the District of Columbia (MSDC) was deemed guilty of racial discrimination by the US Senate when it denied admission to 3 African American physicians between 1869 and 1870. As a result of these exclusionary practices, the National Medical Society of the District of Columbia (NMSDC) was formed. However, in 1870 the AMA, as recommended by their Committee on Ethics, voted to accept the all-white delegation from the MSDC and exclude the integrated NMSDC. The AMA also determined that Howard University violated the AMA Code of Ethics by admitting women to the faculty. Sarah Hackett Stevenson became the first woman admitted into the AMA in 1876.[12,13]

AMA decisions to support discriminatory and exclusionary policies of local and state medical societies contributed to the continued structural racism and inequity that currently persists. Exclusion from medical societies blocked African Americans from gaining hospital privileges, board certification, and career advancement.[12]

Medical societies other than the AMA were formed to provide a voice and fulfill the needs of URM physicians and patients. The National Medical Association, the forerunner of these organizations, was founded in 1895, as an all-inclusive organization to serve the interests of African American physicians and patients. The American Women's Medical Association was founded in 1915 and the National Hispanic Medical Association in 1994. The oldest medical association in America, the APA, was founded in 1844. The APA had similar historical struggles in addressing the needs of URM psychiatrists and marginalized underrepresented patients. See **Fig. 1** for a timeline of important APA historical events that contributed to the frustration and determination of its black members to fight for equity.[13,14]

The Black Psychiatrists of America (BPA) addressed systemic societal issues of African Americans affecting mental health and organizational obstacles encountered by black psychiatrists. Its Executive Committee was charged to present their demands to the APA Board of Trustees meeting in May 1969 and confront their professional medical organization on the issues of civil rights, inequities, and legal and ethical issues of racism. As a result, the number of black psychiatrists in decision-making positions increased; the BPA Executive Committee was made an APA committee; and the BPA was instrumental in negotiations for having a minority center within the National Institute of Mental Health.[15,16] Today, the APA has made progress over time through its initiatives and policies.[17]

More recent efforts by organized medicine to address past discriminatory practices and improve health equity have attempted to increase recruitment of URMs in medicine and psychiatry. Beginning in 1969, the Association of American Colleges (AAMC)

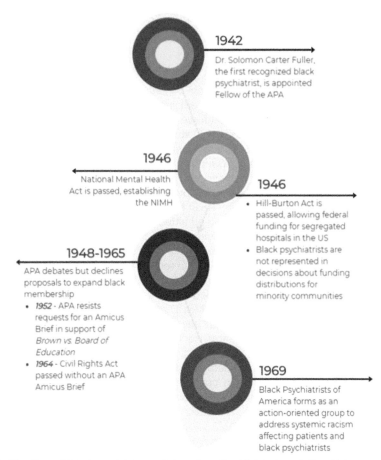

Fig. 1. Timeline of black psychiatry and American Psychiatric Association history.

worked to increase URMs in medicine. In 2007, the AAMC recommended the process of "holistic review"[18] of applicants after legal challenges, including a 2003 US Supreme Court ruling that "racial balancing" of admissions was unconstitutional. Holistic review is a process of selection based on the whole applicant—personal attributes, life experiences, and academic performance. This mission-based, legally compliant approach is applied in the screening, interview, and selection process. Despite the recommended use of holistic reviews, the number of URMS has not increased significantly in medicine, or psychiatry, specifically.

RECRUITMENT CHALLENGES

One barrier to the recruitment of URMs is an incomplete use of holistic reviews. For example, training programs commonly require a minimal score and no failures on the United States Medical Licensing Examination for residency interview selection. Applicants to fellowship programs may be screened by annual in-service examination scores, and many fellowship applicants volunteer these scores on resumes or during interviews. Some faculty believe test performance is the sole measure of medical knowledge. Accreditation standards that track graduate board pass rates accelerate the emphasis on scores. Programs and applicants with limited resources may not have the capacity to improve test and board preparation with costly test-taking specialists or board preparation courses, often placing URM candidates at a disadvantage. Further complicating the adoption of holistic reviews is the time commitment required. Most selection committee members are volunteers with little protected time. Clarification of areas of potential concern on applications requires time and processes that may not be available even if an applicant would add value to a program.

Unconscious/implicit bias (ie, learned stereotypes that are automatic and unintentional that can influence behavior) affects recruitment during screening, interviewing, and selection. Unconscious/implicit bias training has been implemented in many academic institutions as a means of meeting accreditation requirements for diversity and inclusion. The quality of such training varies, which affects effectiveness. Faculty involved in recruitment must examine personal, program, departmental, and institutional biases, with a focus on solutions, not blame, to increase the numbers of URMs and address health disparities. Self-reflection and introspection are part of life-long learning, professional development, and personal growth. Modeling such practices contributes to an environment of acceptance, inclusion, and support for students, residents, and faculty. Faculty demonstrating the ability to engage in difficult conversations for students, residents, and faculty may help them tolerate strong negative reactions when examining personal attitudes, feelings, and beliefs.

SUPERVISION OF UNDERREPRESENTED IN MEDICINE PHYSICIANS

Supervision and mentoring, regardless of who comprises the dyad, must occur in a trusting relationship to be effective. What happens when difficult issues, such as microaggressions, discrimination, or bigotry, must be discussed in supervision? Both supervisor or trainee may feel unequipped to manage such issues and thus avoid further discussion. The supervisor or learner may deny anything happened or may feel unheard or dismissed and therefore, not bring up such difficult topics again; the result can be an erosion of trust and less effective supervision.

Faculty supervisors may have training to manage a "difficult" learner, but do they train regarding possible intangible causes of the difficulties for such a learner? A URM learner may have trouble learning due to microaggressions, feeling like they do not belong, must defend everything they do, like they are scrutinized more, and that they must work twice as hard as their peers to be seen as half as good. Such issues are corrosive to self-esteem and self-confidence, perpetuating the cycle of poor performance and negative evaluations, depression, and anxiety.[19] These intangible topics are discussed among URM learners but less often with faculty or non-URM learners for fear of being negatively labeled or fear of retaliation.[20]

Lack of diversity in faculty and perceived "treatment" of URM faculty in training environments contribute to challenges of recruitment,[21] retention, and supervision of URM trainees. Future initiatives to address mental health equity and training a culturally competent psychiatric workforce will need to address supporting URM faculty.

EDUCATION INITIATIVES IN SUPPORT OF MENTAL HEALTH EQUITY
Cultural Competency

Accreditation Council for Graduate Medical Education (ACGME) requirements for psychiatry support cultural competence in 4 of the 6 general medical competencies. In *Patient Care,* residents must evaluate, treat, and develop a therapeutic alliance with patients and families from diverse backgrounds. Residents must have *Medical Knowledge* about sociocultural, ethnic, and religious/spiritual factors, as well as gender and sexual orientation that influence physical and psychological development. Residents need to understand American culture and subcultures including immigrant populations, particularly those found in the patient community associated with the educational program. Learning should focus on the cultural elements of the relationship between the resident and the patient, including the dynamics of differences in cultural identity, values and preferences, and power. Residents are expected to develop *Communication Skills* that facilitate effective communication with patients and families across a broad range of socioeconomic and cultural backgrounds, including work with interpreters. In *Professionalism*, residents must demonstrate sensitivity and responsiveness to a diverse patient population, including but not limited to, diversity in gender, age, culture, race, religion, disabilities, and sexual orientation[22]; however, in Milestones 2.0, which will be implemented in 2021, this language was moved to the new Supplemental Guide.[23]

Unfortunately, there has been little consensus about what cultural competency training entails, and so educators have implemented heterogeneous education interventions. Early cultural competency teaching models focused on knowledge about the characteristics of particular cultural groups. These interventions ranged from celebrations of various festivals and providing typical foods of a specific cultural group to learning traits about how mental health is perceived or reasons why particular patients from a cultural group do not adhere to treatment recommendations to unusual presentations of mental health disorders in a cultural group (culture-bound syndromes).[24] Elements of these interventions may assist trainees in understanding their patients, but concerns have been raised that this pedagogy may promote stereotypes amid increasing recognition that individual patients from a cultural group may not identify with characteristics ascribed to that group and that patients may identify with greater or lesser intensity to a multiplicity of intersectional identities based on ethnicity, gender, race, and sexual orientation, among others.[25]

Cultural Humility

In contrast, the concept of *cultural humility* recognizes that culture is unique to individuals and that providers must understand their personal culture and the beliefs they bring to a patient encounter.[26] The concept of humility is based on the idea that the more one is exposed to patients from different cultures, the more one recognizes the challenge of knowing how any particular patient identifies.[27] The Outline for Cultural Formulation (OCF), included in the DSM-IV, an attempt to incorporate anthropological concepts into psychiatry, was criticized for not providing sufficient guidance to clinicians. The Cultural Formulation Interview (CFI), part of DSM-5, standardized questions that can be used by clinicians working with patients. The CFI starts with broad questions about the patient's presenting concerns and definition of the problem; subsequent questions probe and use the patient's idiom of distress.[28]

Recent Cultural Education Interventions in Psychiatry Residency Training

There is modest evidence that education improves cultural competence in general psychiatry residents. A 9-week multicultural competence curriculum based on the OCF found improvements in residents' multicultural knowledge, skills, and attitudes.[29] Another 12-week cultural competence course based on the CFI has been described but cultural competence outcomes were not measured.[30] In another study, psychiatry residents at 6 programs had a 1-hour resident-led didactic session to introduce the CFI and completed pre- and postintervention questionnaires. During the didactic, participants also reflected on their own cultural identity and discussed their identity in pairs and in a large group. Analysis demonstrated a significant improvement in self-perceived cultural competency as measured by pre- and posttest scores.[31] Recently a promising case-based curriculum has been published to explicate fundamental concepts in cultural psychiatry.[32] A helpful toolkit for psychiatry resident training in cultural competence has also been published.[22]

Structural Competency

ACGME requirements for psychiatry *Systems-Based Practice* require that residents must assist patients in dealing with system complexities and disparities in mental health resources. The concept of *structural competency* promotes a shift from pedagogies that emphasize a cross-cultural understanding of patients to pedagogies that emphasize forces that influence health outcomes at levels higher than individual interactions.[33] Social and structural determinants of health—including, but not limited to, race, gender, culture, income, education, immigration, neighborhood environment, economic forces, and public policies—collectively contribute more to health and well-being than the totality of health care services.[34] Recognizing the important role that social determinants play in the health of individuals living in communities, structural competency trains providers to understand that symptoms of illness and health behaviors such as adherence may represent the downstream implications of structural decisions such as zoning laws, urban and rural infrastructures, and policing policies in those communities.[33]

Structural Competency Education Interventions in Psychiatry Residency Education

Although there have been calls for psychiatry training programs to implement required structural competency education to graduate physicians who act on structural determinants of mental health,[35] most interventions are electives. The Structural Vulnerability Interview provides a structured set of questions that trainees can learn to use[36]; data from this interview can be used to develop a Structural Formulation to explain symptoms and health behaviors. A casebook describing structural competency interventions has been published,[37] but few programs have addressed outcome measures. A group of educators, residents, and community members have published a set of experiential educational interventions that form a required curriculum in structural competency for psychiatry residents at Yale.[38–40] Although these interventions were well received overall, only 60% of residents who participated reported having used a structural competency perspective in their own clinical work. The hope that such educational interventions will develop knowledge about structural topics and foster critical thinking skills that residents will use in their future work with patients requires further evaluation. It may be that a structural competency perspective must be developed during medical school when trainees are establishing their approach to patient care and reinforced in residency.

Advocacy

When residents understand the role that social structures play in creating health disparities, they want to change these structures. Training residents to be advocates allows them to use their expertise and influence to advance the health and well-being of individual patients, communities, and populations.[41] Advocacy is an ACGME subcompetency under *Systems-Based Practice*, specifically to "advocate for quality patient care and optimal patient care systems." The issue of what perspective to take on deciding whether a patient care system is optimized is not addressed in the requirement. The perspective matters, as the results of "system optimization," would likely be quite different if the optimization is from the perspective of an individual patient, the physician, the institution, the community, or underserved minority communities. In fact, "system optimization" could be the rationale to terminate programs to improve health disparities among minority communities.

Advocacy Education in Psychiatry Residency Training

An APA resource document provides an excellent overview of the role of psychiatrists as advocates and reviews 7 psychiatry residency programs advocacy curricula, many initiated by residents.[42] Most curricula contained both didactic and experiential components; in at least 4 programs the advocacy curriculum is a component of the formal curriculum. Many of the programs invite special speakers, including legislators, community activists, and journalists to offer perspectives and answer questions. Although there are no outcome studies of the effect of an advocacy curriculum in psychiatry residents, 5 years after participating in an advocacy curriculum in a pediatrics residency, pediatricians were more engaged in community activities than their peers who did not participate.[43]

TRAINING IN CHILD AND ADOLESCENT PSYCHIATRY AND MENTAL HEALTH EQUITY

Child and adolescent psychiatry (CAP) is a relative late-comer to the world of academic psychiatry; its first certifying examinations were administered in 1959. From its community-based, multidisciplinary, psychosocial foundation in the Child Guidance movement of the 1920s to 1950s, including an emphasis on trauma, poverty, and other social determinants, CAP strove in the 1980s and 1990s to develop medical legitimacy; in 1983, the American Academy of Child and Adolescent Psychiatry (AACAP) called for an evidence-based approach in "Child Psychiatry: A Plan for the Coming Decades," and CAP research grew.[44] Reimbursement patterns and legislative changes that first required, and then incentivized, the study of medication safety and efficacy in pediatric patients resulted in increased demand for child psychiatry services. Today virtually all states have significant CAP shortages, and the pediatric population is underserved.

Broadly, CAP training is often distinguished by its emphasis on development and family, educational, and community-based systems. However, development from infancy through adolescence, a traditional part of CAP didactic curricula, when conventionally taught reflects the white European male bias of other academic areas of study. With notable exceptions (eg, Ainsworth, Klein, and Anna Freud), major developmental theorists—Piaget, Erikson, Winnicott—were European men who studied primarily white subjects and extrapolated from that experience. Gilligan's In A Different Voice uncovered the implicit gender bias in Kohlberg's theory of moral development.[45] The historic binary conceptualization of male/female gender development has given way to a range of gender identities and sexual orientations, although acceptance of these differences varies significantly across cultures.

More recent research on child development explores more deeply potential racial, cultural, and other biases. For example, global studies of attachment over 30 years across socioeconomic classes, racial, and ethnic groups have found bias to be a universal phenomenon but with differing rates of insecure attachment across cultures. Different child-rearing practices and values across cultures influence attachment, parenting patterns, and goals of development.[46] Developmental goals such as "self-regulation" and "separation and individuation" are normative in Western culture but not in some Asian cultures.[47] The role of adverse childhood events, acculturative stress, and intersectionality is only now being more fully recognized as critical in identity formation and mental health in youth.

Similarly, certain diagnostic categories, comorbidities, treatments, and avenues to care in childhood and adolescence have been recognized as potential areas for implicit bias. For example, growing evidence suggests that nonwhite minorities in the United States are more likely to receive a diagnosis of disruptive behavior disorder than attention-deficit hyperactivity disorder (ADHD).[48] Similarly, higher rates of antipsychotic use in children in foster care have been documented, even after controlling for demographic and diagnostic factors.[49] Screening instruments and psychological testing used to diagnose learning disorders and depression may or may not be cross-culturally normed.[46,50] Disorders of glucose metabolism in young patients with first-episode psychosis are often attributed to antipsychotic medication; however, evidence suggests that both "visible minority status" and childhood trauma are more likely to be associated with elevated HbA1c levels at baseline.[51] Barriers to accessing care for children of immigrants and racial minorities persist.[52] When minority youth are in treatment of disorders such as depression, ADHD, or traumatic brain injury, they are more likely to receive lower quality and less consistent care.[53–55]

The system in which training occurs promotes a "hidden curriculum" around issues of diversity, equity, and inclusion that has persisted despite ever-evolving changes in national demographics. URMs in psychiatry have not increased significantly from 2012 to 2017, with blacks remaining at 6.2% to 7.0% of total psychiatry residents and Latinx residents at 7.1% to 8.0%; they are believed to be even more underrepresented in child psychiatry.[56] Women typically outnumber men in CAP fellowship (60.7% women vs 39.3% men, averaged 2012–17; APA 2018), but gender inequity in opportunity, pay, and promotion persists.[57,58] Requirements from accreditation bodies, such as ACGME's new diversity requirement (ACGME 2019), policies such as the American Academy of Pediatrics' Diversity and Inclusion Statement, and resources such as AACAP's "Diversity and Cultural Competency Curriculum for Child and Adolescent Psychiatry Training" may help to shape the direction of training programs in these areas.[59–61]

TRAINING PRACTICES TO ACHIEVE MENTAL HEALTH EQUITY

In addition to practices previously described, the authors believe that steps could be taken by regulatory agencies such as the ACGME, the American Board of Psychiatry and Neurology (ABPN), and state medical boards to further affect mental health equity. These agencies have a powerful influence on psychiatric education and the continuing education of board-certified practitioners.

During residency training, the ACGME could specify that training in the history of psychiatry links the contributions that biased diagnoses and unequal treatment to mental health inequity so that residents can appreciate the contribution of such practices to past wrongs. Education about biases (rather than training to "remove" biases) should be mandatory, and quality improvement should include activities such as advocacy experiences and meetings with community panels and partners about their needs and experiences with accessing mental health care. Requirements for training residents to work with community groups, schools, local law enforcement, and faith-based communities that interface with their patient population may also have an impact.

Additional educational materials that would enhance education in such areas could include developing Observed Structured Clinical Encounters for students and residents to provide practice in approaching patients with cultural humility and structural competency. Role-play supervision scenarios for faculty development could facilitate the often-difficult discussions about race, gender, and power that lead to problematic encounters with trainees. The American Association of Directors of Psychiatry Residency Training (AADPRT), Association of Directors of Medical Student Education in

Psychiatry, and AACAP, among others, could produce such curricula through initiatives within the diversity, inclusion, and equity committees of their respective organizations and disseminate them among their members.

Following graduation, continuing education and maintenance of certification requirements specified by state boards and the ABPN should include a requirement for training about social determinants of health and advocacy. This would parallel similar requirements for quality improvement or opioid prescribing.

As discussed earlier, whom we train is equally important as how we train. Therefore, the authors recommend that institutional commitments to diversity (with measurable outcomes) be a part of the Clinical Learning Environment Review visit of the ACGME and the Liaison Committee on Medical Education requirements for residency and fellowship programs and medical schools. Because this requirement is often extremely challenging, there should be templates available for how it may be achieved. Finally, realistic parameters should be set for examination scores and effective remediation approaches disseminated to accommodate students who may be at a disadvantage taking standardized tests or who have had less access to science, technology, engineering, and mathematics curricula in secondary school and college.

SUMMARY

This article has briefly summarized several major drivers of mental health inequity in adults and children. Biases in psychiatric diagnosis and treatment, structural racism in recruitment, and inadequate faculty development efforts to acknowledge and moderate biases remain, despite efforts to improve. Cultural and structural competency and advocacy training interventions, along with requirements for such training in practicing psychiatrists, may have an impact. More robust enforcement of diversity standards may influence needed institutional change.

DISCLOSURE

Dr D.M. Sudak receives book royalties from American Psychiatric Press, WILEY and Wolters-Kluver and payment in kind from the American Association of Directors of Psychiatric Residency Training (AADPRT). Dr S.M. DeJong receives book royalties from Elsevier and payment in kind from the American Association of Directors of Psychiatric Residency Training (AADPRT), the American College of Psychiatrists (ACP), the APA, and the AACAP. Dr B. Bailey receives payment in kind from the American Psychiatric Association and the ACGME. Dr R.M. Rohrbaugh receives book royalties from Radcliffe and Routledge Publishers.

REFERENCES

1. Goodell W. The American slave code in theory and practice shown by its statutes, judicial decisions and illustrative facts. Third edition. NY: American and Foreign Anti-Slavery Society; 1853. Archive.org. Available at: https://archive.org/details/americanslavecod00lcgood/page/86. Accessed August 1, 2019.
2. Alsan M, Wanamaker M. Tuskegee and the Health of Black Men. Q J Econ 2018; 115(3):715–53.
3. Metzl J. The protest psychosis: how schizophrenia became a black disease, 30. Boston: Beacon Press; 2009. p. 95–107.
4. Gara MA, Minsky S, Silverstein SM, et al. A Naturalistic Study of Racial Disparities in Diagnosis and an Outpatient Behavioral Health Clinic. Psychiatr Serv 2019; 70(2):130–4.

5. Segal SP, Bola JR, Watson MA. Race, quality of care, and antipsychotic prescribing practices in psychiatric emergency services. Psychiatr Serv 1996;47(3): 282–6.
6. McGuire TG, Miranda J. Racial and Ethnic Disparities in Mental Health Care: Evidence and Policy Implications. Health Aff (Millwood) 2008;27(2):393–403.
7. Bharata VS, Gupta A, Brokenleg M. The Hiawatha Asylum for Insane Indians: The First Federal Mental Health Hospital for an Ethnic Group. Am J Psychiatry 1999; 156:767.
8. Yellowbird P. Wild Indians: Native Perspectives of the Hiawatha Asylum for Insane Indians. MindFreedomInternational.org. 2001. Available at: https://mindfreedom. org/wp-content/uploads/attachments/wild-indians.pdf. Accessed November 1, 2019.
9. National Academies of Sciences, Engineering and Medicine. Communities in action: pathways to health equity. Washington, DC: The National Academies Press; 2017. Available at: https://doi.org/10.17226/24624/. Accessed August 1, 2019.
10. Aguilar-Gaxiola S, Loera G, Méndez I, et al. Community-defined solutions for Latino mental health care disparities: California reducing disparities project, Latino strategic planning workgroup population report. Sacramento (CA): UC Davis; 2012.
11. American Psychiatric Association Council on Minority Mental Health and Health Disparities. APA Official Actions: Position statement on resolution against racism and racial discrimination and their adverse impacts on mental health 2018. Available at: https://www.psychiatry.org/File%20Library/About-APA/Organization-Documents-Policies/Policies/Position-2018-Resolution-Against-Racism-and-Racial-Discrimination.pdf. Accessed December 13, 2019.
12. AMA History of Medicine. The American Medical Association and race. Chicago: AMA; 2014. Available at: 10.1001/virtualmentor.2014.16.6.mhst1-1406. Accessed December 13, 2019.
13. Baker RB, Washington HA, Olakanmi O, et al. African American physicians and organized medicine, 1846-1968: Origins of a racial divide. JAMA 2008;300(3): 306–13.
14. American Psychiatric Association. Library and archives. Available at: https://www. psychiatry.org/psychiatrists/search-directories-databases/library-and-archive. Accessed April 8, 2020.
15. Pierce CM. Black psychiatry one year after Miami. J Natl Med Assoc 1970;62(6): 471–3.
16. Wille CV, Kramer BM, Brown BS. Racism and mental health: Essays. Pittsburgh (PA): University of Pittsburgh; 1973.
17. American Psychiatric Association. Diversity & health equity. 2019. Available at: https://www.psychiatry.org/psychiatrists/cultural-competency. Accessed December 14, 2019.
18. Association of American Medical Colleges. Holistic Review. 2020. Available at: https://www.aamc.org/services/member-capacity-building/holistic-review. Accessed December 13, 2019.
19. Cokley K, Smith L, Bernard D, et al. Impostor feelings as a moderator and mediator of the relationship between perceived discrimination and mental health among racial/ethnic minority college students. J Couns Psychol 2017;64(2): 141–54.
20. Osseo-Asare A, Balasuriya L, Huot SJ, et al. Minority resident physicians' views on the role of race/ethnicity in their training experiences in the workplace. JAMA Netw Open 2018;1(5):e182723.

21. Pierre JM, Mahr F, Carter A, et al. Underrepresented in medicine recruitment: Rationale, challenges, and strategies for increasing diversity in psychiatry residency programs. Acad Psychiatry 2017;41(2):226–32.
22. Corral I, Johnson TL, Shelton PG, et al. Psychiatry Resident Training in Cultural Competence: An educator's toolkit. Psychiatr Q 2017;88:295–306.
23. Accreditation Council for Graduate Medical Education. Supplemental Guide: Psychiatry. 2020. Available at: https://www.acgme.org/Portals/0/PDFs/Milestones/PsychiatrySupplementalGuide.pdf?ver=2020-03-10-161139-047. Accessed April 21, 2010.
24. Aggarwal N, Cedeno K, Guarnaccia P, et al. The meanings of cultural competence in mental health: an exploratory focus group study with patients, clinicians, and administrators. Springerplus 2016;5:384–97.
25. Powell Sears K. Improving cultural competence education: the utility of an intersectional framework. Med Educ 2012;46:545–51.
26. Tervalon M, Murray-Garcia J. Cultural Humility versus Cultural Competence: A critical distinction in defining physician training outcomes in multicultural education. J Health Care Poor Underserved 1998;9:117–25.
27. Yaeger K, Bauer-Wu S. Cultural Humility: Essential foundation for clinical researchers. Appl Nurs Res 2013;26:251–6.
28. Aggarwal N, Nicasio A, Desilva R, et al. Barriers to implementing the DSM5 cultural formulation interview: a qualitative study. Cult Med Psychiatry 2013;37:505–33.
29. Harris TL, McQuery J, Raab B, et al. Multicultural psychiatric education: using the DSM-IV TR Outline for Cultural Formulation to improve resident cultural competence. Acad Psychiatry 2008;32:306–12.
30. Aggarwal N, Desilva R. Developing cultural competence in health care professions: a fresh approach. Med Educ 2013;47:1143–4.
31. Mills S, Xiao AQ, Wolitzky-Taylor K, et al. Training on the DSM-5 Cultural Formulation Interview Improves Cultural Competence in General Psychiatry Residents: A Multi-Site Study. Acad Psychiatry 2016;40:829–34.
32. Trinh NT, Chen JA. Sociocultural issues in psychiatry: a casebook and curriculum. New York: Oxford Press; 2019.
33. Metzl J, Hansen H. Structural Competency: Theorizing a new medical engagement with stigma and inequality. Soc Sci Med 2014;103:126–33.
34. Braveman P, Gottlieb I. The Social Determinants of Health: it's time to consider the causes of the causes. Public Health Rep 2014;129(Suppl 2):19–31.
35. Hansen H, Braslow J, Rohrbaugh RM. From Cultural to Structural Competency-Training Psychiatry Residents to Act on Social Determinants of Health and Institutional Racism. JAMA Psychiatry 2018;75:117–8.
36. Bourgois P, Holmes SM, Sue K, et al. Structural Vulnerability: Operationalizing the Concept to Address Health Disparities in Clinical Care. Acad Med 2017;92:299–307.
37. Hansen H, Metzl J, editors. Structural competency in mental health and medicine. Cham (Switzerland): Springer Nature Switzerland AG; 2019.
38. Bromage W, Encandela J, Cranford M, et al. Understanding Health Disparities through the Eyes of Community Members: A Structural Competency Education Intervention. Acad Psychiatry 2019;43:244–7.
39. Mathis W, Cyrus K, Jordan A, et al. Introducing a Structural Competency Framework for Psychiatry Residents: Drawing Your Neighborhood. Acad Psychiatry 2019;43:635–8.

---

40. Rohrbaugh RM, Bromage W, Spell V, et al. Allying with Our Neighbors to Teach Structural Competence: The Yale Department of Psychiatry Structural Competency Community Initiative. In: Hansen H, Metzl J, editors. Structural competency in mental health and medicine. Cham (Switzerland): Springer Nature Switzerland AG; 2019. p. 159–66.

41. Frank JR. The CanMEDS 2005 physician competency framework. Ottowa, ON: Office of Education, The Royal College of Physicians and Surgeons of Canada; 2005.

42. Kennedy K, Vance MC. PDF download of APA resource document: advocacy teaching in psychiatry residency training programs. Washington, DC: American Psych Assoc; 2017.

43. Minkovitz CS, Goldshore M, Solomon BS, et al, Community Pediatrics Training Initiative Workgroup. Five-year follow-up of community pediatrics training initiative. Pediatrics 2014;134(1):83–90.

44. Hoagwood KE, Jensen PS, Acri MC, et al. Outcome domains in child mental health research since 1996: Have they changed and why does it matter? J Am Acad Child Adolesc Psychiatry 2012;51:1241–60.e2.

45. Gilligan C. In a different voice. Cambridge (MA): Harvard University Press; 1982.

46. Davies D. Child development - a practitioners guide. 3rd edition. New York: The Guilford Press; 2011.

47. Haight W. The pragmatics of caregiver-child pretending at home: Understanding culturally specific socialization practices. In: Goncu A, editor. Children's engagement in the world: sociocultural perspectives. New York: Cambridge University Press; 1999. p. 128–47.

48. Fadus MC, Gosmbirg KR, Sobowale K, et al. Unconscious bias and the diagnosis of disruptive behavior disorders and ADHD in African American and Hispanic Youth. Acad Psychiatry 2020;44:95–102.

49. Vanderwerker L, Akincigil A, Olfson M, et al. Foster care, externalizing disorders, and antipsychotic use among Medicaid-enrolled youth. Psychiatr Serv 2014;65: 1281–4.

50. Mellick W, Hatkevich C, Venta A, et al. Measurement invariance of depression symptom ratings across African American, Hispanic/Latino, and Caucasian adolescent psychiatric inpatients. Psychol Assess 2019;31:833–8.

51. Veru-Lesmes F, Rho A, King S, et al. Social determinants of health and preclinical glycemic control in newly diagnosed first-episode psychosis patients. Can J Psychiatry 2018;63:547–56.

52. Georgiades K, Paksarian D, Rudolph KE, et al. Prevalence of mental disorder and service use by immigrant generation and race/ethnicity among US adolescents. J Am Acad Child Adolesc Psychiatry 2018;57:280–7.

53. Cummings JR, Ji X, Lally C, et al. Racial and ethnic differences in minimally adequate depression care among Medicaid-enrolled youth. J Am Acad Child Adolesc Psychiatry 2019;58:128–38.

54. Ji X, Druss BG, Lally C, et al. Racial-ethnic differences in patterns of discontinuous medication treatment among Medicaid-insured youths with ADHD. Psychiatr Serv 2018;1:322–31.

55. Moore M, Jimenez N, Graves JM, et al. Racial disparities in outpatient mental health service use among children hospitalized for traumatic brain injury. J Head Trauma Rehabil 2018;33:177–84.

56. American Psychiatric Association. 2018 Resident-Fellow Census. Available at: https://www.psychiatry.org/residents-medical-students/medical-students/resident-fellow-census. Accessed April 17, 2020.

57. Petrovic-Dovat L, Forgey Borlik M, Wadell P, et al. Bridging the gender and diversity gap: Mentorship models for addressing underrepresentation of women psychiatrists. Special Interest Study Group 5 presented at American Academy of Child and Adolescent Psychiatry Annual Meeting. Chicago, IL, October 18, 2019.
58. Frellick M. Physician salaries up in 2019; report shows who earns the most. Medscape Psychiatry 2019. Available at: https://www.medscape.com/viewarticle/911668#vp_2. Accessed April 17, 2020.
59. Accreditation Council of Graduate Medical Education (ACGME). Common Program Requirements (Residency), 1.C. 2019. Available at: https://www.acgme.org/Portals/0/PFAssets/ProgramRequirements/CPRResidency2019.pdf. Accessed April 17, 2020.
60. American Academy of Pediatrics. AAP Diversity and Inclusion Statement. Pediatrics 2018;141(4):e20180193.
61. American Academy of Child and Adolescent Psychiatry. Diversity and cultural competency curriculum for CAP training. 2011. Available at: https://www.aacap.org/App_Themes/AACAP/Docs/resource_centers/cultural_diversity/Diversity_and_Cultural_Competency_Curriculum_for_CAP_Training.pdf. Accessed April 17, 2020.

Improving Research Quality to Achieve Mental Health Equity

Quianta Moore, MD, JD[a],*, Patrick S. Tennant, PhD, MS[a],
Lisa R. Fortuna, MD, MPH[b]

KEYWORDS

- Mental health • Research • Equity • Disparities
- Community-based participatory research (CBPR) • Human-centered design (HCD)

KEY POINTS

- Inequities that exist throughout our society are also present and influential in medical and mental health research, where they can become embedded and self-perpetuating.
- Current and historical inequities in the mental health research process are one cause of persistent disparities in mental health services and outcomes.
- Full inclusion (with decision-making authority) of previously disempowered groups is needed to redress the disparities in the mental health system.
- A framework for more equitable research to practice pipeline through the use of community-based participatory research and human-centered design is proposed.

INTRODUCTION

The historic and current inequities in mental health are complex and multifaceted. Equity is a concept that acknowledges systemic and societal barriers to achieving health and wellness. The Robert Wood Johnson Foundation defines health equity as every person having "a fair and just opportunity to be as healthy as possible."[1] This definition frames health in terms of equal opportunity to be healthy, as opposed to simply the outcome of health. The implicit declaration of this framing—that not only are we not all equally healthy, but we do not all have an equal opportunity to be healthy—is critical in addressing mental health equity.

[a] Center for Health and Biosciences, Rice University's Baker Institute for Public Policy, 6100 Main Street, MS-40, PO Box 1892, Houston, TX 77251-1892, USA; [b] Zuckerberg San Francisco General Hospital and Trauma Center, University of California San Francisco, 1001 Potrero Avenue, 7M16, UCSF Campus Box 0852, San Francisco, CA 94110, USA
* Corresponding author.
E-mail address: qm4@rice.edu
Twitter: @QuiantaMoore (Q.M.); @Tennant_PS (P.S.T.); @fortuna_lisa (L.R.F.)

Psychiatr Clin N Am 43 (2020) 569–582
https://doi.org/10.1016/j.psc.2020.05.005
0193-953X/20/© 2020 Elsevier Inc. All rights reserved.

psych.theclinics.com

Abbreviations	
CBPR	Community-based participatory research
HCD	Human-centered design
SODH	Social determinants of health

A HISTORY OF INEQUITIES

The opportunity to be healthy is influenced by social circumstances rooted in race, immigration status, political, economic, and neighborhood factors. The health care system is not siloed from the rest of society. The same factors that influence an individual's access to other opportunities, such as a good education and economic security, influence an individual's access to opportunities to be as healthy as possible. In fact, decades of research demonstrate that social, environmental, and economic factors have a greater impact on health outcomes than clinical care, with 80% of health outcomes attributed to these social determinants of health (SODH).[2] SDOH, defined by the Centers for Disease Control and Prevention as "conditions in the places where people live, learn, work, and play," are influenced by the distribution of money, power, and resources at the individual, community, and national levels.[3] SDOH influence all health outcomes, including negative mental health outcomes.[4]

Owing to historic racial and ethnic discrimination, minority populations are more likely to experience negative SDOH and are also more likely to distrust the health care system.[5] Distrust of health care further disadvantages minority populations in that they do not receive needed medical care[6] and are not included in the research to develop the evidence for clinical interventions.

A critical, reflective review of the participation and contribution of the health care field to adverse conditions and community mistrust is necessary as a first step toward achieving equity. We focus our inequity discussion on race because the social construct of race compounds and perpetuates disadvantage in the United States, and racial disparities exist in every outcome of individual and community well-being.[7] Moreover, much of the knowledge and advances in medicine are a result of unethical medical experimentation on racial minorities. We use the treatment of African Americans as an illustrative example because of the unique role African Americans have played in US history. For instance, in the 1820s and 1830s a former slave, John Brown, describes being routinely burned and "bled" by a prominent physician to identify the thickness of black skin.[5(p54)] A hundred years later, inhumane research on black patients continued with crude lobotomies performed on African American children as young as 6 years who were determined to be "aggressive" or "hyperactive."[5] Lobotomies were used to make African American boys and prisoners more "docile," and as part of a National Institute of Mental Health–funded project to "cure" urban rioters in the 1960s. As recently as the late 1990s, an institutional review board–approved study injected African American boys who had an older sibling in juvenile detention with the drug fenfluramine to determine if there was a genetic basis for aggressive or violent behavior. Not only was the study scientifically flawed, but the treatment of the children was unethical and inhumane. Additionally, fenfluramine was not approved for use in children at the time of the study, and was banned by the Food and Drug Administration in 1997.[5] Moreover, false beliefs about African Americans persist today. A study published in 2016 revealed that 50% of white medical students and residents surveyed held false beliefs about African Americans, including the belief that black skin is thicker.[8] Additionally, the stigmatization of African Americans as violent or more aggressive remains pervasive.[9]

IMPLICIT BIAS

Although the acceptability of overt racism is less prevalent today, the remnants of racism and false beliefs prevail through implicit bias and contribute to inequities in health care delivery. The term implicit bias refers to attitudes, beliefs, and stereotypes that unintentionally influence behaviors, decisions, and actions.[10] Research demonstrates that the majority of health care providers have a negative implicit bias against marginalized groups.[11] Implicit bias can harm the health of socially disadvantaged communities. For example, racial and ethnic minorities experience suboptimal care from service providers owing to negative implicit bias.[10,12] This circumstance can cause a reluctance to seek treatment,[13] or a lesser likelihood of receiving a proper assessment or the appropriate treatment.[14,15] Mental health systems are particularly vulnerable to the negative impacts of implicit bias because the diagnosis and treatment of mental health conditions rely heavily on provider discretion.[10] For instance, higher rates of schizophrenia diagnoses in African Americans may be due to providers attributing and weighting observations differently for different racial groups,[16] thereby attributing pathology to patient behavior or characteristics when in reality the "symptoms" noted are cultural differences within a normal spectrum.[17]

Implicit bias is a major contributor to health disparities,[18] which are the differences in health outcomes between population groups, particularly when there is worse health among the socially disadvantaged group.[19] Health disparities are the product of inequity, and substantial disparities exist in mental health outcomes. For example, persistence of diagnosis (ie, the continuation or recurrence of a disorder across at least 2 years) is higher among African Americans and Latinx people than in whites and suicide rates are higher in American Indian and Alaskan Native young adults than in all other racial and ethnic groups.[20,21]

The disparities in rates of mental health outcomes are, unfortunately, paired with disparities in mental health service access, which has also been documented in many conditions for a multitude of vulnerable groups.[22] Adverse disparities in the provision of mental health services exist for racial and ethnic minorities,[23] pregnant women,[24] low-income populations,[25] and those in certain US states.[26] For example, Latinx children and youth are more likely than their white counterparts to have unmet needs for mental health services.[25]

Moving forward, health delivery organizations must acknowledge their history and develop systems that ensure no one is disadvantaged from achieving mental wellness because of societal position or any other socially defined context, resulting in an equal opportunity to be healthy.[27] Intentionally addressing systemic implicit bias within the system is required to overcome historical and systemic barriers to accessing quality care for vulnerable populations.

THE PATH FORWARD

The first step in ensuring an equitable path forward is to create equal access to opportunities to participate in the research that drives clinical practice. Developing interventions that improve mental health for everyone is critical to achieving equity, but there are often challenges in recruiting communities who have been historically mistreated by the medical field. Without the inclusion of socially disadvantaged populations, we have a research-to-practice pipeline that inadequately understands, and thus inadequately treats, groups of people who are not included in the research and practice foundations of the mental health field. Moreover, inequities are perpetuated in the research processes and the epistemologic frames on which they are based. Inequities can also shape who is included in the research used to inform treatments. For example, Lally and colleagues[28] conducted a retrospective analysis of a study sample intended to be representative of a population of individuals with severe mental illness and found that eligible individuals who did not participate in the study reported poorer mental health status at the time of eligibility than individuals who did participate. Not including those with worse mental health status results in therapies for severe mental illness that may not be effective for the entire population of individuals with severe mental illness. Similar disparities in the likelihood an individual was contacted, consented, or participated in studies have been found for other subgroups (ie, age and ethnicity,[29] ethnicity,[30] intellectual ability,[31] neurocognitive and social functioning[32]). The effects of these disparities are then multiplied when researchers and clinicians use those biased findings as a basis for designing and implementing treatments. Excluded groups end up with therapies that are not as effective as they could be, and patients and their families spend resources on suboptimal treatments, creating an additional financial burden. Additionally, ineffective health care validates community mistrust and further increases health disparities, thus contributing to a pernicious cycle of increasing separation in the opportunity for optimal health between advantaged and disadvantaged groups. Thus, we need an inclusive research-to-practice pipeline that accounts for historical and present-day inequities by addressing barriers, and reshapes the systematic processes of the health care system.

Partnering with Communities

A decrease in health disparities can be used to measure how close we are to achieving systemic equity in health care, and necessitates a deeper understanding and appreciation for the barriers that have decreased opportunities for socially disadvantaged groups. The populations who are at a social disadvantage are best positioned to inform and educate health care providers as to how to decrease barriers and increase opportunities for health. Moreover, developing partnerships with community members allows providers and researchers to work against bias. Community-based participatory research (CBPR) is an approach to research that includes community members in the process of influencing health services quality improvement efforts, identifying research questions and promoting innovation in intervention and study design[33] to improve community health and reduce health disparities.[34] A CBPR approach requires a partnership with community members, which results in sharing power, resources, credit, results, and knowledge between communities and researchers.[35] There is a reciprocal appreciation of each partner's knowledge and skills at each stage of the project, including problem definition, issue selection, research design, conducting research, interpreting the results, and determining how the results should be used for action. Because CBPR is an orientation to research, this approach can be used with any research design or methodology.[36] For instance, CBPR has increasingly been used in randomized clinical controlled trials.[37] Rather than the traditional approach to research, which prioritizes academic or clinical research priorities to advance a general body of knowledge or test a clinical intervention, CBPR is an iterative process. It seeks to incorporate research, reflection, and action in a cyclical process to consider the applicability of the research in addressing community-relevant problems or tailoring interventions to cultural and community contexts.[35] For example, a CBPR approach was used in a research project with parents of children with emotional disturbance from the formative phase (to identify the research focus) to the codesigning phase (to implement a provider–parent communication intervention).[38] Similarly, a CBPR approach was used to adapt an evidence-based intervention for Latinx people with chronic disease and co-occurring minor depression to identify implementation barriers and to tailor the intervention for community settings.[39]

A persistent challenge encountered by the scientific field, especially in mental health, is the ability to include those individuals and populations who may be the most marginalized and voiceless.[40] Many of these individuals have limited access to medical research and evidence-based treatments because of factors such as their living conditions, homelessness, foster care, displacement, immigration status, or a combination of intersecting minority status and identities.[41] For example, researchers have noted that many of the scientifically proven post-traumatic stress disorder treatments have not reached rural veterans owing to stigma and geographic barriers.[42] CBPR has been used to address the issue of participation in research trials by hard-to-reach populations to move toward equitable participation in research[40] and has been used to incorporate the voices of communities in research, particularly around health disparities.[43]

Leveraging Community Expertise

Similar to CBPR, human-centered design (HCD) acknowledges the principle that community members are experts in their own right and are best positioned to inform the solution.[43] HCD uses a process of iterative systems-based changes and continuous input from the end-user to design the most useable interventions.[44,45] HCD emerged from the fields of computer science and artificial intelligence and focuses on how to create the most innovative or creative solutions to community or "human" problems. HCD has 3 distinct phases for problem solving: the inspiration phase, the ideation phase, and the implementation phase.[46] The inspiration phase is focused on building empathy within the design team for individual lived experiences.[47] The goal is to better understand the intended users of the product, potential barriers, and workaround solutions people have created.[47] The ideation phase engages intended users to generate ideas on how to solve the identified problem.[47] During the implementation phase, the design team creates low-fidelity prototypes to test broad concepts, which allows end-users to provide feedback on the potential solution.[47] HCD is primarily applied to technological innovations and has been used in the mental health field to design the best ways to use and implement technology-based interventions in low-resource settings.[44] Technological or digital delivery interventions need an evidence base that is contextual and relevant to the target population,[42] and HCD could be an approach to gaining an understanding of how diverse populations engage with and use these technologies, and what individuals find most accessible and useful.[44] Overall, HCD has the potential to be a tool in social innovation, and HCD strategies can help to reach hard-to-reach populations, thereby achieving broad impact and scale.[46]

A NEW INTEGRATED APPROACH

Approaches that empower communities and individuals to drive their own behavioral health care can improve engagement and can help to decrease health inequities. CBPR and HCD both create processes and strategies for identifying problems and developing solutions through cocreation and bidirectional knowledge sharing. However, there are differences in the values, purpose, and process of each that, if combined, could yield even more advancement for equitable research and practice. For example, in a study designed to understand and address youth violence disparities in Latinx youth, a CBPR approach was used to engage and empower youth to collect data, plan community forums, recruit participants, and use Photovoice.[43,48] HCD methods were used to foster creativity and idea generation, taking the youth from identifying the problem to cocreating solutions.[43] The integrated CBPR and HCD approach allowed researchers to identify negative contributors to youth mental health and well-being, as well as created an opportunity for the community to generate future-centered solutions.[43]

Although HCD has traditionally been used in the private sector, combining HCD strategies with CBPR helps research to equitably move along the research-to-practice pipeline by equipping researchers with the tools needed to ensure the community voice is incorporated at every stage. Research using these approaches has sought to shift clinical practice by engaging community members on using their voice to participate in clinical decision making with their health care providers.[49,50] This shift in the research and medical practice paradigm requires that mental health providers have support and training on how to be receptive to shared power in decision making with patients, and to understand how patient empowerment facilitates therapeutic alliance and improves care.[49,50] Thus, before engaging in community participatory efforts, it is necessary for health care providers to understand that partnering with patients in clinical and research decision making not only encourages patients to improve their health, but also limits the impact of potential harms from providers and systemic biases.

Community members are best positioned to identify challenges in achieving optimal health and wellness for their communities, as well as to codevelop solutions. The National Institute of Health's Roadmap and the Clinical Translational Science Award program, as well as the practice-based research networks, have recognized the value of participatory research and its potential for producing stronger research that is more responsive and relevant to community needs than traditional research models.[51] However, health care practitioners have to be supported in accepting a new model of practice that includes sharing power with patients and communities to achieve optimal outcomes. The first step is to imbed implicit bias trainings throughout the medical education process and provide continuing education credits for professionals to attend these trainings.

Implicit bias training of health care providers is necessary to reach the goal of a more equitable health care system.[52] Although cultural competence trainings are often cited as a possible solution, they have mixed effectiveness in improving patient outcomes and often focus on explicit bias by recognizing and accepting cultural differences.[53] Implicit bias trainings, in contrast, aim to remove and replace automatic, implicit, and subconscious attitudes and beliefs through various mechanisms, including counterstereotypes.[52] Because negative implicit biases are malleable, they can be changed with intervention. For instance, studies evaluating the impact of repeated trainings to denounce stereotypes and replace them with counterstereotypes resulted in a decrease in stereotype activation.[52] No research has been conducted to date on the impact of implicit bias reduction on patient outcomes, but we postulate that addressing the root cause of a major contributor to health disparities will yield improved patient outcomes.

Moreover, financial incentives for hospitals and providers to adopt implicit bias trainings as a requirement for staff and clinicians will yield a greater widespread adoption of nondiscriminatory practices. Research demonstrates that social consensus can dismantle subconscious stereotypes and can decrease discriminatory behavior.[52] Thus, if health care systems adopt a supportive culture of recognizing bias and making intentional efforts to reduce negative beliefs and behaviors, provider motivation to change could increase.[52]

A PRACTICAL MODEL FOR EQUITABLE RESEARCH

Once health care systems and providers do the internal, reflective work necessary to engage community members in a culturally sensitive manner, an integrated CBPR and

Table 1
Steps to integrating CBPR and HCD for equitable research

Step 1: Identify population or community of focus	Hospital systems are required to conduct a community needs assessment, which could help to identify the population of focus (ie, the patient population for whom the greatest health disparities are present). Individual or group practices can review patient records and conduct a data analysis to identify the population of focus or subgroups that show differential outcomes in quality of care measures. Traditional CBPR methods do not often provide guidance on "who" the community is or who the population of focus should be. In contrast, HCD uses an approach of intentionally selecting extremes within a targeted population to elicit a diversity of opinions and experiences. For example, if a study involves those with substance abuse challenges, the population of focus would consist of those with extreme differences in number of years using (ie, beginner and $\geq$20 years), and have a variety of demographic attributes, beliefs, and behavioral attitudes, with an over-representation for hard-to-reach groups. Ensuring inclusivity and recognizing diversity within populations is important for advancing equity, and leveraging the strengths of HCD in step one aids in capturing the voices of everyone.
Step 2: Build relationships with community or patient leaders	Although some providers or hospital systems have the bandwidth to conduct community outreach, smaller, less-resourced practices can identify patients in their practice who are civically engaged, and who would be willing to be a bridge between the community and the health care provider. Whereas HCD focuses less on relationship-building, CBPR is a process that prioritizes long-term relationships and trust with community partners to shift power from researchers to communities.[46] Examples of relationship building could be attending community meetings, bringing food to meetings, volunteering to participate in a community event or activity, and making financial investments in the community (ie, hiring community members as research staff, purchasing research supplies from businesses within the community). Smaller practices could also engage with the community around issues that the patient leader has identified as important. Relationship building is key to effective participation and engagement in the research process.

(continued on next page)

Table 1 (continued)	
Step 3: Community engagement	Community or patient leaders can leverage their networks and relationships to facilitate community member participation in meetings to identify a common agenda between the health care system and the community, and key barriers and assets to achieving improved mental health and well-being. Strategies and guiding principles from HCD can be used throughout the community engagement process (ie, no wrong ideas, collaboration, inclusion, innovation, iteration).[47]
Step 4: Develop research questions and design	Although clinicians and researchers have the expertise to determine the best methodology and research design to answer the research questions of interest, research questions should be codeveloped with community members. Moreover, with the appropriate training, community members can be engaged in the research process, including survey design and administration, data collection, PhotoVoice, focus groups, and project implementation. Funds should be included in grant budgets to ensure community members are compensated for their work, and community members should be considered a valuable part of the research team. Although HCD encourages a transdisciplinary team across sectors, the members consist mostly of experts. A CBPR approach includes community members as part of the research team and values the expertise they bring to the project.[46]
Step 5: Data analysis and interpretation	Data can tell a story about a community or population and the storytellers are frequently researchers or medical professionals. Implicit bias often colors how socially disadvantaged communities are depicted in the narrative and CBPR shifts the paradigm, giving community members the right to inform what story is being told about them and to provide context to researchers to better understand the findings.[54] Although there are some concerns that community involvement may bias results,[55] systemic reviews and meta-analyses demonstrate that CBPR may strengthen the internal and external validity of research.[37]
Step 6: Implementation and scaling of interventions	Although CBPR has strengths in ensuring equitable dissemination of research results and identifying structural and organizational factors that need to be addressed, HCD approaches are more helpful in creating tangible products or services that can be rapidly tested and adjusted with continuous input from the end-user. The implementation phase of HCD requires the design team to define its success and develop a plan for monitoring and evaluating implementation.[47] Integrating this phase with CBPR principles would create opportunities for community members to cocreate definitions of success and the rapid cycle evaluation plan.

(continued on next page)

Table 1 (continued)	
Step 7: Accountability	CBPR principles encourage accountability to the community. A community advisory board is one strategy for ensuring accountability to the community from the beginning to end of the research-to-practice pipeline. A community advisory board can be set up at any time throughout the research-to-practice continuum, but should definitely be in existence by the end of the project to ensure accountability to the values and agreed upon principles of the community-health care partnership. Identifying CAB members is important and incorporating the values of HCD to include a diversity of perspectives will enhance the CAB's impact.

HCD approach that draws from the strengths of both can be used in the steps in **Table 1** to ensure that medical care is effective for the communities they serve.

Although the steps in Table 1 are proposed linearly, some projects or initiatives may begin at the implementation or accountability stage (**Fig. 1**). Additionally, the steps presented could also be used in health services innovation projects that are not considered to be typical research projects, such as quality improvement. Regardless, steps 1 and 2 are critical to improving mental health equity and reducing health disparities, and therefore should be the initial component of any initiative or project.

OPPORTUNITIES FOR INNOVATION AND IMPLEMENTATION

This proposed model of research can be used to examine and improve the impact of promising, field-wide changes, such as technology-supported interventions and

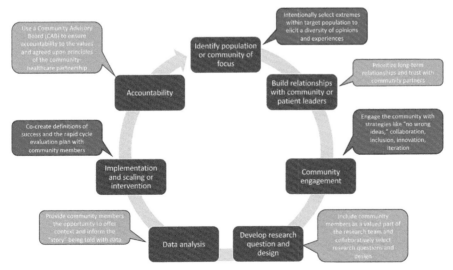

Fig. 1. The cycle of equitable research, informed by CBPR and HCD. CBPR strategies are depicted in *green* and HCD strategies are depicted in *red*.

integrated behavioral health care, on mental health equity. For example, the application of technology in the coordination and delivery of mental health services holds substantial potential for improving equity,[56,57] but that potential has yet to be fully realized and complications remain.[58,59] Researchers who integrate the principles of CBPR and HCD in the development, implementation, and evaluation of these mental health technologies will be better prepared to identify and respond to barriers to mental health that are not addressed by (or are created by) the use of these technologies. Similarly, the integration of behavioral health into primary care settings has already been shown to decrease disparities in access to services for African Americans and outcomes for Latinx people,[60,61] but concerns about the appropriateness of primary care physicians assessing and treating mental health disorders remain and more research is needed.[62] Using the model and approaches proposed here can ensure that research efforts incorporate the populations for whom integrated behavioral health is designed to serve. Fully integrated care is an especially promising health care system intervention because it often includes efforts to address both mental health and the SODH within the primary care setting. Given the inherent complexity and interdependence of integrating mental and physical health care with social factors, particularly for groups with complex social circumstances,[63] the community perspective is critical to a successful intervention. Researchers and health care systems must include the community perspective throughout the process to achieve mental health equity.

SUMMARY

The model we propose aims to provide guidance on how the integration of evidence-based participatory research approaches, CBPR and HCD, can help to remove inequities and barriers in the research-to-practice pipeline and help to correct mistaken assumptions and biases that underlie many behavioral health interventions.[64] By including community articulated needs, priorities, and recommendations we resist replicating existing service disparities in our clinical and research practice, thereby optimizing opportunities for socially disadvantaged populations to achieve mental health and well-being.[64]

DISCLOSURE

The authors have nothing to disclose.

REFERENCES

1. What is health equity? RWJF. 2017. Available at: https://www.rwjf.org/en/library/research/2017/05/what-is-health-equity-.html. Accessed December 16, 2019.
2. Hood CM, Gennuso KP, Swain GR, et al. County health rankings: relationships between determinant factors and health outcomes. Am J Prev Med 2016;50(2): 129–35.
3. Social Determinants of Health | CDC. 2019. Available at: https://www.cdc.gov/socialdeterminants/index.htm. Accessed December 16, 2019.
4. Allen J, Balfour R, Bell R, et al. Social determinants of mental health. Int Rev Psychiatry 2014;26(4):392–407.
5. Washington H. Medical apartheid: the dark history of medical experimentation on Black Americans from the colonial times to the present. Harlem Moon 2006. Available at: https://www.penguinrandomhouse.com/books/185986/medical-apartheid-by-harriet-a-washington/. Accessed December 11, 2019.

6. New Study Reveals Lack of Access as Root Cause for Mental Health Crisis in America. National Council. Available at: https://www.thenationalcouncil.org/press-releases/new-study-reveals-lack-of-access-as-root-cause-for-mental-health-crisis-in-america/. Accessed December 16, 2019.

7. Wolff T, Minkler M, Wolfe S, et al. Collaborating for equity and justice: moving beyond collective impact. Nonprofit Quarterly. 2017. Available at: https://nonprofitquarterly.org/collaborating-equity-justice-moving-beyond-collective-impact/. Accessed December 16, 2019.

8. Hoffman KM, Trawalter S, Axt JR, et al. Racial bias in pain assessment and treatment recommendations, and false beliefs about biological differences between blacks and whites. Proc Natl Acad Sci U S A 2016;113(16):4296–301.

9. Oliver MB. African American men as "criminal and dangerous": implications of media portrayals of crime on the "criminalization" of African American men. J Afr Am Stud (New Brunsw) 2003;7(2):3–18.

10. Merino Y, Adams L, Hall WJ. Implicit bias and mental health professionals: priorities and directions for research. Psychiatr Serv 2018;69(6):723–5.

11. Hall WJ, Chapman MV, Lee KM, et al. Implicit racial/ethnic bias among health care professionals and its influence on health care outcomes: a systematic review. Am J Public Health 2015;105(12):e60–76.

12. Jones AL, Cochran SD, Leibowitz A, et al. Racial, ethnic, and nativity differences in mental health visits to primary care and specialty mental health providers: analysis of the medical expenditures panel survey, 2010-2015. Healthc Basel Switz 2018;6(2). https://doi.org/10.3390/healthcare6020029.

13. Roberts AL, Gilman SE, Breslau J, et al. Race/ethnic differences in exposure to traumatic events, development of post-traumatic stress disorder, and treatment-seeking for post-traumatic stress disorder in the United States. Psychol Med 2011;41(1):71–83.

14. Charron E, Francis EC, Heavner-Sullivan SF, et al. Disparities in access to mental health services among patients hospitalized for deliberate drug overdose. Psychiatr Serv 2019;70(9):758–64.

15. Stein BD, Dick AW, Sorbero M, et al. A population-based examination of trends and disparities in medication treatment for opioid use disorders among Medicaid enrollees. Subst Abuse 2018;39(4):419–25.

16. Trierweiler SJ, Neighbors HW, Munday C, et al. Clinician attributions associated with the diagnosis of schizophrenia in African American and non-African American patients. J Consult Clin Psychol 2000;68(1):171.

17. Earl TR, Fortuna LR, Gao S, et al. An exploration of how psychotic-like symptoms are experienced, endorsed, and understood from the National Latino and Asian American Study and National Survey of American Life. Ethn Health 2015;20(3): 273–92.

18. Smedly BD, Stith AY, Nelson AR. Unequal treatment: confronting racial and ethnic disparities in health care. Institute of Medicine of the National Academies; 2003. Available at: http://www.nationalacademies.org/hmd/Reports/2002/Unequal-Treatment-Confronting-Racial-and-Ethnic-Disparities-in-Health-Care.aspx. Accessed December 16, 2019.

19. Braveman P. What are health disparities and health equity? we need to be clear. Public Health Rep 2014;129(Suppl 2):5.

20. Breslau J, Kendler KS, Su M, et al. Lifetime risk and persistence of psychiatric disorders across ethnic groups in the United States. Psychol Med 2005;35(3): 317–27.

21. Jiang C, Mitran A, Minino A, et al. Racial and gender disparities in suicide among young adults aged 18–24: United States, 2009–2013 2015. Available at: https://www.cdc.gov/nchs/data/hestat/suicide/racial_and_gender_2009_2013.htm. Accessed December 16, 2019.
22. Office of the Surgeon General (US), Center for Mental Health Services (US), National Institute of Mental Health (US). Mental health: culture, race, and ethnicity: a supplement to mental health: a report of the surgeon general. Rockville (MD): Substance Abuse and Mental Health Services Administration (US); 2001. Available at: http://www.ncbi.nlm.nih.gov/books/NBK44243/. Accessed December 16, 2019.
23. Cook BL, Trinh N-H, Li Z, et al. Trends in racial-ethnic disparities in access to mental health care, 2004–2012. Psychiatr Serv 2017;68(1):9–16.
24. Weinreb L, Byatt N, Moore Simas TA, et al. What happens to mental health treatment during pregnancy? Women's experience with prescribing providers. Psychiatr Q 2014;85(3):349–55.
25. Kataoka SH, Zhang L, Wells KB. Unmet need for mental health care among U.S. children: variation by ethnicity and insurance status. Am J Psychiatry 2002;159(9):1548–55.
26. Sturm R, Ringel JS, Andreyeva T. Geographic disparities in children's mental health care. Pediatrics 2003;112(4):e308.
27. McNulty M, Smith JD, Villamar J, et al. Implementation research methodologies for achieving scientific equity and health equity. Ethn Dis 2019;29:10.
28. Lally J, Watkins R, Nash S, et al. The representativeness of participants with severe mental illness in a psychosocial clinical trial. Front Psychiatry 2018;9. https://doi.org/10.3389/fpsyt.2018.00654.
29. Patel R, Oduola S, Callard F, et al. What proportion of patients with psychosis is willing to take part in research? A mental health electronic case register analysis. BMJ Open 2017;7(3):e013113.
30. Jackson JS, Torres M, Caldwell CH, et al. The National Survey of American Life: a study of racial, ethnic and cultural influences on mental disorders and mental health. Int J Methods Psychiatr Res 2004;13(4):196–207.
31. Russell G, Mandy W, Elliott D, et al. Selection bias on intellectual ability in autism research: a cross-sectional review and meta-analysis. Mol Autism 2019;10(1):9.
32. Piskulic D, Addington J, Auther A, et al. Using the global functioning social and role scales in a first-episode sample. Early Interv Psychiatry 2011;5(3):219–23.
33. Wilson E, Kenny A, Dickson-Swift V. Ethical challenges in community-based participatory research: a scoping review. Qual Health Res 2018;28(2):189–99.
34. Wallerstein N, Duran B, Oetzel J, et al. Community-based participatory research for health: advancing social and health equity. 3rd edition. Josey-Bass; 2017. Available at: https://www.wiley.com/en-us/Community+Based+Participatory+Research+for+Health%3A+Advancing+Social+and+Health+Equity%2C+3rd+Edition-p-9781119258858. Accessed December 16, 2019.
35. Wallerstein N, Duran B. The conceptual, historical and practical roots of community based participatory research and related participatory traditions. In: Minkler M, Wallerstein N, editors. Community-based participatory research for health. San Francisco: Jossey-Bass; 2003. p. 27–52.
36. Buchanan DR, Miller FG, Wallerstein N. Ethical issues in community-based participatory research: balancing rigorous research with community participation in community intervention studies. Prog Community Health Partnersh 2007;1(2):153–60.

37. Collins SE, Clifasefi SL, Stanton J, et al. Community-based participatory research (CBPR): towards equitable involvement of community in psychology research. Am Psychol 2018;73(7):884–98.
38. Unertl KM, Schaefbauer CL, Campbell TR, et al. Integrating community-based participatory research and informatics approaches to improve the engagement and health of underserved populations. J Am Med Inform Assoc 2016;23(1):60–73.
39. Aguado Loi CX, Alfonso ML, Chan I, et al. Application of mixed-methods design in community-engaged research: lessons learned from an evidence-based intervention for Latinos with chronic illness and minor depression. Eval Program Plann 2017;63:29–38.
40. Bonevski B, Randell M, Paul C, et al. Reaching the hard-to-reach: a systematic review of strategies for improving health and medical research with socially disadvantaged groups. BMC Med Res Methodol 2014;14(1):42.
41. Israel BA, Schulz AJ, Parker EA, et al. Review of community-based research: assessing partnership approaches to improve public health. Annu Rev Public Health 1998;19(1):173–202.
42. Fortney JC, Pyne JM, Kimbrell TA, et al. Telemedicine-based collaborative care for posttraumatic stress disorder: a randomized clinical trial. JAMA Psychiatry 2015;72(1):58.
43. Kia-Keating M, Capous D, Liu S, et al. Using community based participatory research and human centered design to address violence-related health disparities among Latino/a youth. Fam Community Health 2017;40(2):160–9.
44. Lyon AR, Munson SA, Renn BN, et al. Use of human-centered design to improve implementation of evidence-based psychotherapies in low-resource communities: protocol for studies applying a framework to assess usability. JMIR Res Protoc 2019;8(10):e14990.
45. Lyon AR, Koerner K. User-centered design for psychosocial intervention development and implementation. Clin Psychol (New York) 2016;23(2):180–200.
46. Chen E, Leos C, Kowitt SD, et al. Enhancing community-based participatory research through human-centered design strategies. Health Promot Pract 2019. https://doi.org/10.1177/1524839919850557. 1524839919850557.
47. The field guide to human-centered design: design kit. San Francisco (CA): IDEO; 2015.
48. Wang C, Burris MA. Photovoice: concept, methodology, and use for participatory needs assessment. Health Educ Behav 1997;24(3):369–87.
49. Alegría M, Polo A, Gao S, et al. Evaluation of a patient activation and empowerment intervention in mental health care. Med Care 2008;46(3):247–56.
50. Alegría M, Carson N, Flores M, et al. Activation, self-management, engagement, and retention in behavioral health care: a randomized clinical trial of the DECIDE intervention. JAMA Psychiatry 2014;71(5):557–65.
51. Schmittdiel JA, Grumbach K, Selby JV. System-based participatory research in health care: an approach for sustainable translational research and quality improvement. Ann Fam Med 2010;8(3):256–9.
52. Matthew DB. Just medicine: a cure for racial inequality in American health care. New York: New York University Press; 2015.
53. Lie DA, Lee-Rey E, Gomez A, et al. Does cultural competency training of health professionals improve patient outcomes? A systematic review and proposed algorithm for future research. J Gen Intern Med 2011;26(3):317–25.

54. Hsu C, Cruz S, Placzek H, et al. Patient perspectives on addressing social needs in primary care using a screening and resource referral intervention. J Gen Intern Med 2019. https://doi.org/10.1007/s11606-019-05397-6.
55. Resnik DB, Kennedy CE. Balancing scientific and community interests in community-based participatory research. Account Res 2010;17(4):198–210.
56. McGregor B, Mack D, Wrenn G, et al. Improving service coordination and reducing mental health disparities through adoption of electronic health records. Psychiatr Serv 2015;66(9):985–7.
57. Benavides-Vaello S, Strode A, Sheeran BC. Using technology in the delivery of mental health and substance abuse treatment in rural communities: a review. J Behav Health Serv Res 2013;40(1):111–20.
58. Ralston AL, Andrews AR, Hope DA. Fulfilling the promise of mental health technology to reduce public health disparities: review and research agenda. Clin Psychol Sci Pract 2019;26(1):e12277.
59. López CM, Qanungo S, Jenkins C, et al. Technology as a means to address disparities in mental health research: a guide to "tele-tailoring" your research methods. Prof Psychol Res Pr 2018;49(1):57–64.
60. Ayalon L, Areán PA, Linkins K, et al. Integration of mental health services into primary care overcomes ethnic disparities in access to mental health services between black and white elderly. Am J Geriatr Psychiatry 2007;15(10):906–12.
61. Bridges AJ, Andrews AR, Villalobos BT, et al. Does integrated behavioral health care reduce mental health disparities for Latinos? initial findings. J Lat Psychol 2014;2(1):37–53.
62. Possemato K, Johnson EM, Beehler GP, et al. Patient outcomes associated with primary care behavioral health services: a systematic review. Gen Hosp Psychiatry 2018;53:1–11.
63. Holden K, McGregor B, Thandi P, et al. Toward culturally centered integrative care for addressing mental health disparities among ethnic minorities. Psychol Serv 2014;11(4):357–68.
64. Alegría M, Alvarez K, Ishikawa RZ, et al. Removing obstacles to eliminating racial and ethnic disparities in behavioral health care. Health Aff (Millwood) 2016;35(6):991–9.

Moving?

Make sure your subscription moves with you!

To notify us of your new address, find your **Clinics Account Number** (located on your mailing label above your name), and contact customer service at:

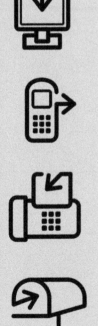

Email: journalscustomerservice-usa@elsevier.com

800-654-2452 (subscribers in the U.S. & Canada)
314-447-8871 (subscribers outside of the U.S. & Canada)

Fax number: 314-447-8029

Elsevier Health Sciences Division
Subscription Customer Service
3251 Riverport Lane
Maryland Heights, MO 63043

*To ensure uninterrupted delivery of your subscription, please notify us at least 4 weeks in advance of move.

Printed and bound by CPI Group (UK) Ltd, Croydon, CR0 4YY

03/10/2024

01040477-0014